Taniguchi Symposia on Brain Sciences No.12

NEURAL PROGRAMMING

Taniguchi Symposia on Brain Sciences No. 12
PROGRAM COMMITTEE

Masao Ito (Chairman), Suguru Arimoto,
Kazuo Sasaki, Jun Tanji

The Taniguchi Foundation, Division of Brain Sciences
ORGANIZING COMMITTEE

Osamu Hayaishi (Chairman)
Osaka Medical College, Takatsuki, Osaka 569, Japan
Masao Ito
Department of Physiology, Faculty of Medicine, University of Tokyo, Tokyo 113, Japan
Yasuji Katsuki
National Institute for Physiological Sciences, Okazaki, Aichi 444, Japan
Yutaka Sano
Department of Anatomy, Kyoto Prefectural University of Medicine, Kyoto 602, Japan
Yasuzo Tsukada
Department of Physiology, School of Medicine, Keio University, Tokyo 160, Japan
Hiroshi Yoshida
Department of Pharmacology, Osaka University Medical School, Osaka 539, Japan
Teruo Nakajima (Secretary General)
Department of Psychiatry, Kyoto Prefectural University of Medicine, Kyoto 602, Japan

Taniguchi Symposia on Brain Sciences No.12

NEURAL PROGRAMMING

Edited by
Masao Ito

JAPAN SCIENTIFIC SOCIETIES PRESS Tokyo
KARGER Basel · München · Paris · London · New York · New Delhi · Bangkok · Singapore · Tokyo · Sydney

Supported in part by the Ministry of Education, Science and Culture under Grant-in-Aid for Publication of Scientific Research Result.

Published jointly by
JAPAN SCIENTIFIC SOCIETIES PRESS
2-10 Hongo, 6-chome, Bunkyo-ku, Tokyo 113, Japan
ISBN 4-7622-3598-9
and
S. KARGER AG
P.O. Box, CH-4009 Basel, Switzerland
ISBN 3-8055-5109-6

Distributed in all areas outside Japan by S. Karger AG.

Printed in Japan

PREFACE AND SYNOPSIS

MASAO ITO

Department of Physiology, Faculty of Medicine, University of Tokyo, Tokyo 113, Japan

WHAT IS NEURAL PROGRAMMING?

For a computer, a program is a description of procedures used to generate serial instructions for its operation. When we perform complex motions and behaviors, our brains must be operating according to something similar to such a set of instructions which may be described as a neural program. For example, upon deciding to walk, complex locomotor movements commence immediately and can be maintained without conscious concern about our legs actually moving. A motor program may be defined as a set of muscle commands that are structured before a movement sequence begins, and that allow the entire sequence to be carried out uninfluenced by peripheral feedback (*8*). A motor program may consist of subprograms which have various levels of complexity, down to reflexes, while several motor programs would constitute an over-all motor plan (*3*). A behavioral program may mean a set of movement command similarly structured and executed. For example, various behaviors such as feeding, fleeing, or attacking can be triggered by electric stimulation of a hypothalamic region, as if a tape recording of a behavioral program has been turned on. Neural programming may thus mean the formation of a motor or behavioral program in the brain. Some neural programs are equipped genetically, while others are acquired through learning.

It seems important, however, to point out the vagueness inherent in this definition of neural programming. In fact, all kinds of organized operation of the brain may be regarded as programmed within structures of neuronal networks and neural systems of the brain (*10*). Thus, the entire mechanistic features of the brain's capabilities may be described in terms of neural programming. Neural programming in this wider sense was the major theme of the 12th Taniguchi Foundation Symposium. As a record of the symposium, this book attempts to comprehend recent advances, both experimental and theoretical, in our understanding of the organized operation of the brain at the levels of neuronal networks and neural systems in relation to various types of movement and behavior.

WHERE IS NEURAL PROGRAMMING RUN IN THE BRAIN?

Based on behavioral analyses, it has been assumed that motor programming is performed in a hierarchical manner throughout a number of brain regions. An important task of neuroscience is to reveal functional localization in the brain dedicated to the formation of neural programs and to specify the contribution by each brain area to neural programming.

Involvement of the cerebral premotor, supplementary motor, and primary motor cortices in motor programming has long been suggested. The importance of the cerebral prefrontal cortex in behavioral programming has also been emphasized. Chapters 1–5 address questions as to what sort of neural programming is performed there and how. Population vector, self-initiation, set-related activity, delay period activity, and cortical multiple-component organization are major concepts discussed there.

Roles of subcortical structures such as the cerebellum and basal ganglia in neural programming have also been suggested. Chapters 6–10 are devoted to specification of these subcortical contributions to neural programming. The earlier notion that the paravermalinterpositus division of the cerebellum is dedicated to updating the programmed movement in the course of execution, whilc the hemisphere-dentatus division is involved in the programming of movement parameters before movement initiation (*4*, *5*) is now afforded a theoretical ground in Chapter 16.

Highly organized spatial encoding systems for vision would make unique contributions to neural programming. Tectal motor map for saccadic eye movement, parietal cortical processes for smooth pursuit eye movement, and cerebral cortial mechanisms of pictorial memory are discussed in Chapters 11–13.

HOW ARE MECHANISMS OF NEURAL PROGRAMMING IMPLEMENTED IN NEURAL TISSUES?

In each area of the brain, there is an elaborate neural network. Neural programs should be a product of the operation of such a neuronal network. Local networks in the brain are interconnected to form a large-scaled neural system. Neural programs implied in local networks play a role in the organized operation of such a large-scaled neural system. Studies of neural programming are thus concerned with the architecture and operational principles of neuronal networks and neural systems, dedicated specifically to the formation, storage and implementation of neural programs involved in movement and behavior. In Chapters 14–18, theoretical models of neuronal networks and neural systems for neural programming are developed by introducing various new concepts.

Structural and functional details of neuronal networks and neural systems are accumulating. Excitatory and inhibitory neurons have been distinguished, and four additional types of memory elements have been discovered; long-term potentiation (*1*), long-term depression (*6*), sensitization (*7*), and synaptic sprouting (*9*). With these memory elements incorporated, neuronal network models capable of learning can be constructed.

However, another element, a delay element, must also be involved in order to generate a temporal sequence of movement, which is an essential feature of a neural program. With a delay element, a temporal sequence can be encoded in a spatial sequence, and consequently a neural program can be represented in the spatial pattern of organization in a neuronal network (*2*). In spite of the strong theoretical demand, however, no clear evidence is yet available for such a delay element in the brain. A metronome-like timing device would also be useful in sequential execution of a neural program. However, our present ignorance of such a timing device in the neuronal network is another factor that makes our understanding of neural programming mechanisms difficult. It is an important future task to identify delay elements and timing devices of neuronal networks.

FUTURE PERSPECTIVES

In spite of recent remarkable advancements in neuroscience, there are still gaps in our knowledge of brain mechanisms in general. It is still difficult to specify essential relationships between highly complex structures of the brain and subtle brain functions. Neural programming would be a theme which symbolizes this difficulty, yet it is coming close to our reach from both experimental and theoretical sides. While much effort has been devoted to each side, the importance of close cooperation between them is obvious. New design principles for neural programming seem to await discovery through such interdisciplinary cooperation.

REFERENCES

1. Bliss, T.V.P. and Lømo, T. (1973). *J. Physiol. (London)* **232**, 331–356.
2. Braitenberg, V. and Onesto, N. (1962). Proc. 1st Int. Conf. Med. Cybern. Giannini, Naples, pp. 1–19.
3. Brooks, V.B. (1986). In *The Neural Basis of Motor Control*, pp. 7–8. New York/Oxford: Oxford Univ. Press.
4. Eccles, J.C. (1969). In *Information Processing in the Nervous System*, ed. Leibovic, K.N., pp. 245–269. Berlin/Heidelberg/New York: Springer-Verlag.
5. Evarts, E.V. and Thach, W.T. (1969). *Annu. Rev. Physiol.* **31**, 451–498.
6. Ito, M. (1989). *Annu. Rev. Neurosci.* **12**, 85–102.
7. Kandel, E. and Schwartz, J.H. (1982). *Science* **218**, 433–443.

8. Keele, S.W. (1968). *Psychol. Bull.* **70**, 387–403.
9. Tsukahara, N. (1981). *Annu. Rev. Neurosci.* **4**, 351–379.
10. Young, J.Z. (1978). In *Programs of the Brain*, pp. 3–11. Oxford/New York: Oxford Univ. Press.

CONTENTS

Programming in the Visual System

Programming in Neuronal Network and System

MOTOR PROGRAMMING IN THE CEREBRAL CORTEX

1
MOTOR CORTEX AND REACHING

APOSTOLOS P. GEORGOPOULOS

The Philip Bard Laboratories of Neurophysiology, Department of Neuroscience, The Johns Hopkins University, School of Medicine, Baltimore, Maryland 21205, U.S.A.

Reaching out towards objects of interest is very common in the behavioral repertoire of primates. It involves well coordinated and tightly coupled motions at the elbow and shoulder joints (*25*) by which the hand is brought at or near the object of interest. I discuss in this review the functional properties of cells and cell populations in the primate motor cortex, as they relate to the act of reaching. Other reviews have dealt with general aspects of reaching (*2*), the anatomical pathways involved in reaching (*13*), the effects on reaching of brain lesions (*16*), and the visuomotor coordination underlying reaching to visual targets (*3*).

The study of brain mechanisms underlying voluntary reaching was made possible by the development of techniques for recording the activity of single cells in the brain of behaving animals (*19*). This combined behavioral-neurophysiological experiment provides fine grain and a direct tool for the study of brain mechanisms underlying reaching. The posterior parietal cortex was one of the first brain regions to be studied during reaching (*15, 20*). Indeed, the activity of certain cells in areas 5 and 7 was found to change with reaching in the absence of passive somesthetic driving. It is reasonable to suppose that the planning and execution of reaching involves the activation of several brain regions. Visuospatial information may be transmitted from the parietal to the frontal lobe (*13*), and disturbances in visually guided reaching could result from a disconnection between these two lobes (see, for example, refs. *1*, *12*). The main recipients of posterior parietal projections are premotor areas (*13*). These areas seem to project directly to subcortical structures, including the red nucleus (*14*) and the spinal cord (Strick, this meeting) and, therefore, their influence on the motor function need not be exerted exclusively through the motor cortex. Recordings of single cell activity in behaving monkeys have provided valuable information concerning the possible role(s) of these areas in sensory-motor integration, including preparation for and anticipation of movement (see reviews in refs. *27*, *28*).

Porter and Lewis (*23*) studied the activity of motor cortical cells while monkeys reached out and manipulated a handle in front of them. Murphy *et al.* (*22*) investigated the possible relations between motor cortical cell activity and joint motion and electromyographic (EMG) activity in muscles of the forelimb during reaching. There were three main findings of this study. First, no simple relation was observed between single cell activity and the EMG, even when the muscle from which the EMG was recorded was activated by intracortical microstimulation. Second, single cells related to motion about the shoulder or elbow joints behaved similarly in the task, although the motions produced about these joints could be quite different. And third, the discharge of shoulder-related cells seemed to vary systematically with the movement trajectory. These results indicate that the relations between single cell activity in the motor cortex and components (joint rotation, EMG activity) of reaching are complex.

The spatial parameters of a reaching movement are its direction and amplitude. Psychophysical evidence has been presented (*26*) that these two parameters are meaningful with respect to reaching performance by human subjects, and that indeed performance is better in the direction than in the amplitude domain. Work in our laboratory during the past several years has centered on the relations between neuronal activity in the motor cortex and the direction of

2-D and 3-D reaching movements. The results of these studies are summarized below.

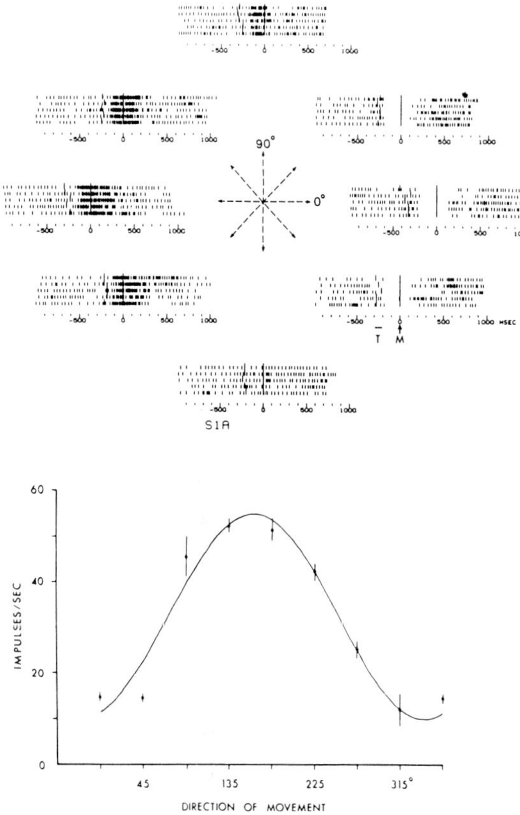

Fig. 1. Directional tuning of a cell recorded in the arm area of motor cortex during 2-D reaching. A: impulse activity during five trials of reaching in the directions indicated in the drawing at the center. Short vertical bars indicate the occurrence of an action potential. Rasters are aligned to the onset of movement (M). Longer vertical bars preceding the onset movement indicate the onset of the target (T); those following the movement indicate, successively, the entrance to the target zone and the delivery of reward. B: average frequency of discharge (±SEM) from the onset of the stimulus until the entry to the target zone are plotted against the direction of movement. Continuous curve is a cosine function fitted to the data using multiple regression analysis. (From ref. *6*, reproduced with permission. Copyright by Society for Neuroscience.)

I. DIRECTIONAL TUNING OF SINGLE MOTOR CORTICAL CELLS

The directional selectivity of motor cortical cells was studied by training rhesus monkeys to point to visual targets in 2-D or 3-D space. In the 2-D experiments monkeys moved an articulated manipulandum towards visual targets on a planar working surface (*6*); in the 3-D studies monkeys reached freely to target buttons (*24*). The electrical signs of activity of single cells in the forelimb area of the contralateral motor cortex were recorded extracellularly while the

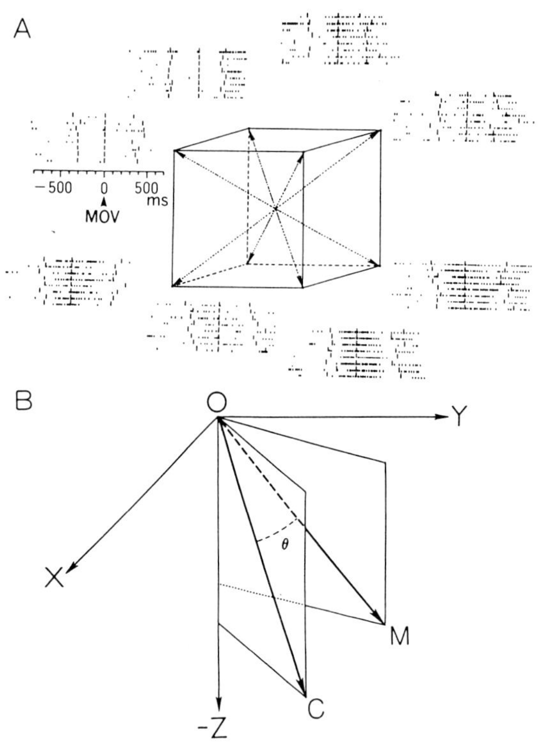

Fig. 2. A: impulse activity of a motor cortical cell during eight equal amplitude movements made from a point in front of the monkey towards eight peripheral targets in 3-D space, as indicated in the drawing at the center; MOV, onset of movement. B: diagram illustrating the general principle of directional tuning. The predicted frequency of cell discharge is a linear function of the cosine of the angle, θ, formed between the direction of movement, M, and the cell's preferred direction, G. (From ref. *11*, reproduced with permission. Copyright by AAAS, 1986.)

monkeys performed the task. The main finding from these studies was that the activity of single motor cortical cells is broadly tuned around a "preferred direction": cell discharge is highest with movements in that direction and decreases gradually with movements made in directions farther and farther away from the preferred one (*6, 11, 24*). This is illustrated in Figs. 1 and 2 for the 2-D and 3-D case, respectively. The directional tuning can be described as a linear function of the cosine of the angle θ formed between the direction of the movement M and the cell's preferred direction C (Fig. 2). The

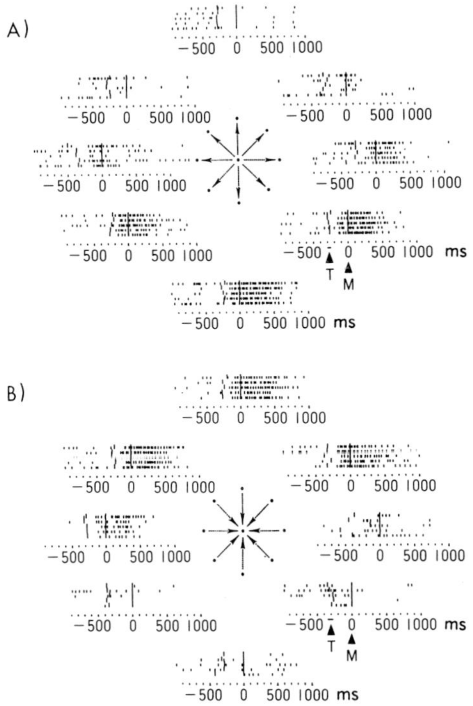

Fig. 3. Cell discharge varies with the direction of movement, not its endpoint. A: impulse activity of a motor cortical cell during five repetitions of eight movements of equal amplitude made from the center of a planar working surface to eight peripheral targets. B: impulse activity of the same cell during movements made from the same peripheral targets towards the same endpoint at the center, as indicated in the diagram at the center. Notice that the discharge varies with the direction of movement, as in A, although all movements terminated in the same endpoint. T, onset of target; M, onset of movement. (From ref. *8*, reproduced with permission by the publisher.)

preferred directions of individual cells differ among cells and range throughout the directional continuum.

In the studies in which monkeys moved from a central point to peripheral points two variables were confounded: the direction of the movement and its endpoint. These variables were dissociated in another series of experiments in which movements were made from the center to several points in a circle but also from points on the circle to its center; in the latter case the direction of the movement varied but its endpoint was the same. It was found that the changes in cell activity were related to the direction of the movement and not its endpoint because they were still present when movements started from various points on a circle but ended in the same point, at the center of the circle (*9*). This is illustrated in Fig. 3.

II. CODING OF THE DIRECTION OF REACHING BY THE NEURONAL POPULATION

The results summarized above indicate that single motor cortical cells are engaged with reaching in different directions throughout 2-D or 3-D space. From this it follows that for a movement in a particular direction, a population of cells with various preferred directions will be active.* How could such a neuronal population encode uniquely a particular direction of reaching? We proposed a code for that problem, first for 2-D reaching (*5*, *8*) and then for 3-D reaching (*10*, *11*). Briefly, the motor cortical command for movement direction can be regarded as the weighted sum of vectorial contributions of individual cells: each cell "votes" in the direction of its preferred direction, and the vote is weighted, for a particular direction or reaching, by the change in cell activity during that movement. The vector sum of these contributions (the "population vector") points in or near the the direction of reaching. Figure 4 illustrates the results obtained for 2-D reaching. Similar results were obtained for 3-D reaching

* Although our recordings of cell activity were performed one at a time, the consistency of the changes in cell activity over time during several repetitions indicates the results would be similar if the recordings were simultaneous. In fact, we have confirmed this assumption by recording simultaneously the activity of motor cortical cells from seven independently movable microelectrodes using the technique described in Mountcastle *et al.* (*21*).

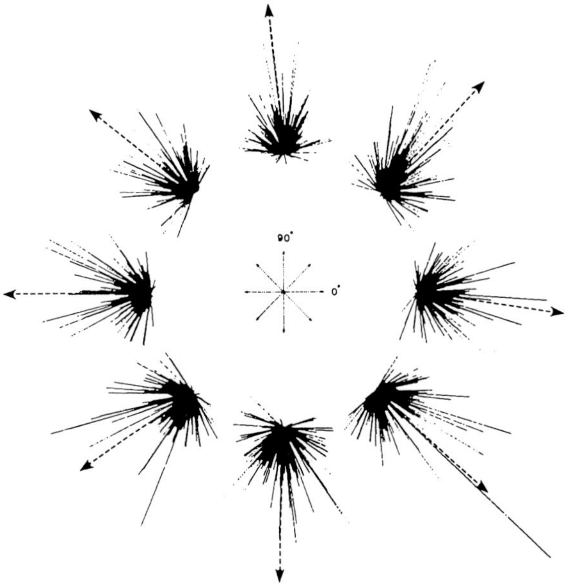

Fig. 4. Population vector analysis applied to eight movement directions in 2-D space. Each cluster represents the same population; the movement directions are shown in the diagram at the center. The population vector (interrupted arrow) points in or near the direction of the movement. (From ref. *5*, reproduced with permission by the publisher.)

(*10, 11*), and even for movements with different points of origin (*18*).

The vectorial representation of directional information at the motor cortical level is a distributed code in the sense that each element (*i.e.*, a neuron) carries only part of the information, whereas the neuronal population determines uniquely the direction of reaching. It is interesting that a population size of about 150–200 cells can provide a good estimate of the direction of the population vector, within 10–15 degrees (*10*). With respect to cortical location, it is noteworthy that neuronal populations in different cortical layers can provide adequate coding for movement direction; for example, the population vectors calculated from cells located in layers II and III or in layers V and VI of the motor cortex both predict well the direction of 2-D reaching (*4*). Given that cells in different layers project to different brain regions (*17*), this finding suggests that the same directional information may be distributed to various brain areas.

III. PREDICTION OF THE DIRECTION OF REACHING DURING THE REACTION TIME AND DURING AN INSTRUCTED DELAY PERIOD

In the tasks used above the animals moved in response to the appearance of a visual target; thus approximately 300 msec, the reaction time, intervened from the onset of the stimulus to the beginning of the movement. It is interesting that the population vector, calculated every 20 msec during the reaction time, predicts well the direction of the upcoming reaching movement. This is illustrated in Fig. 5. Similar results were obtained in the case of movements in 3-D space (*10*). These findings suggest that the population vector is a robust measure of the directional tendency of the neuronal ensemble and that it can serve as a probe to monitor the directionality of the ensemble as time progresses. This became evident when monkeys were trained to withhold the movement for a period of time after the onset of a visual cue signal and to move later

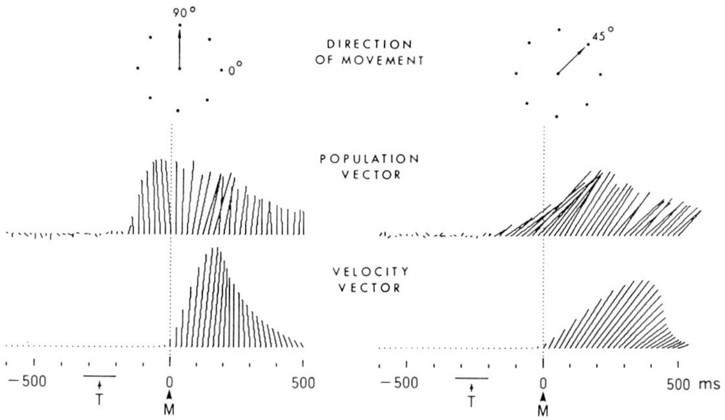

Fig. 5. The population vector points in the direction of movement well before the movement begins. The results for two movement directions in 2-D space are illustrated (top); the population vector was calculated every 20 msec (middle); the average instantaneous (msec bin) velocity of the movement is also shown (bottom). Before the target onset (T), the population vector is very small in length and its direction varies from moment to moment. Well before the onset of movement (M), it increases in length and its direction points to the direction of the upcoming movement. This finding suggests that even the earliest inputs to the motor cortex are relevant to the direction of the upcoming movement. (From ref. *8*, reproduced with permission by the publisher.)

in response to a "go" signal. The population vector computed every 20 msec during this instructed delay period indicated the direction of the movement that was triggered later (7). This suggests that the motor cortex is involved in processing information about the direction of the upcoming movement in space even in the absence of an immediate movement.

SUMMARY

The activity of single cells in the motor cortex is broadly tuned with respect to the direction of reaching, so that the discharge rate is highest with movements in a preferred direction, and decreases progressively with movements made in directions more and more away from the preferred one. Thus the neural command for the direction of reaching can be regarded as an ensemble of cell vectors, with each vector pointing in the cell's preferred direction and having a length proportional to the change in cell activity. The directional outcome of this motor command can be visualized as the vector sum (the "population vector") of the individual cell vectors. This population vector points in the direction of the upcoming movement well before the movement begins and also during an instructed delay period.

Acknowledgement
This work was supported by USPHS Grant NS17413.

REFERENCES

1 Ferro, J.M., Bravo-Marques, J.M., Castro-Caldas, A., and Antunes, L. (1983). *J. Neurol. Neurosurg. Psychiatr.* **46**, 533–539.
2 Georgopoulos, A.P. (1986) *Annu. Rev. Neurosci.* **9**, 147–170.
3 Georgopoulos, A.P. (1989). In *Signal and Sense: Local and Global Order in Perceptual Maps*, ed. Edelman, G.M., Gall, W.E., and Cowan, W.M. New York: John Wiley & Sons, in press.
4 Georgopoulos, A.P. (1989). In *Attention and Performance XIII*, ed. Jeannerod, M., in press.
5 Georgopoulos, A.P., Caminiti, R., Kalaska, J.F., and Massey, J.T. (1983). *Exp. Brain Res.* Suppl. **7**, 327–336.

6 Georgopoulos, A.P., Kalaska, J.F., Caminiti, R., and Massey, J.T. (1982). *J. Neurosci.* **2**, 1527-1537.
7 Georgopoulos, A.P., Crutcher, M.D., and Schwartz, A.B. (1989). *Exp. Brain Res.* **75**, 183-194.
8 Georgopoulos, A.P., Kalaska, J.F., Crutcher, M.D., Caminiti, R., and Massey, J.T. (1984). In *Dynamic Aspects of Neocortical Function*, ed. Edelman, G.M., Gall, W.E., and Cowan, W.M., pp. 501-524. New York; John Wiley & Sons.
9 Georgopoulos, A.P., Kalaska, J.F., and Caminiti, R. (1985). *Exp. Brain Res.* Suppl. **10**, 176-183.
10 Georgopoulos, A.P., Kettner, R.E., and Schwartz, A.B. (1988). *J. Neurosci.* **8**, 2928-2937.
11 Georgopoulos, A.P., Schwartz, A.B., and Kettner, R.E. (1986). *Science* **233**, 1416-1419.
12 Haaxma, R. and Kuypers, H.G.J.M. (1975). *Brain* **98**, 239-260.
13 Humphrey, D.R. (1979). In *Posture and Movement*, ed. Talbott, R.E. and Humphrey, D.R., pp. 51-112. New York: Raven Press.
14 Humphrey, D.R., Gold, R., and Reed, D.J. (1984). *J. Comp. Neurol.* **225**, 75-94.
15 Hyvarinen, J. and Poramen, A. (1974). *Brain* **97**, 673-692.
16 Jeannerod, M. (1986). *Neuropsychologia* **24**, 41-78.
17 Jones, E.G. and Wise, S.P. (1977). *J. Comp. Neurol.* **175**, 391-438.
18 Kettner, R.E., Schwartz, A.B., and Georgopoulos, A.P. (1988) *J. Neurosci.* **8**, 2938-2947.
19 Lemon, R.N. (1984). *Methods for Neuronal Recording in Conscious Animals.* Chichester: John Wiley & Sons.
20 Mountcastle, V.B., Lynch, J .C., Georgopoulos, A.P., Sakata, H., and Acuna, C. (1975). *J. Neurophysiol.* **38**, 871-908.
21 Mountcastle, V.B., Poggio, G.F., Reitbock, H.J., Georgopoulos, A.P., Johnson, K.O., Longerbeam, M.B., Steinmetz, M.A., Phillips, J.R., Brandt, D.K., and Habel, C.G. (1987). *Soc. Neurosci.* Abstr. **13**, 629.
22 Murphy, J.T., Kwan, H.C., MacKay, W.A., and Wong, Y.C. (1982). *Brain Res.* **246**, 141-145.
23 Porter, R. and Lewis, M.Mc. (1975). *Brain Res.* **98**, 21-36.
24 Schwartz, A.B., Kettner, R.E., and Georgopoulos, A.P. (1988). *J. Neurosci.* **8**, 2913-2927.
25 Soechting, J.F. and Lacquaniti, F. (1981). *J. Neurosci.* **1**, 710-720.
26 Soechting, J.F. and Terzuolo, C.A. (1989). In *Attention and Performance XIII*, ed. Jeannerod, M., in press.
27 Tanji, J. (1984). *TINS* **7**, 282-285.
28 Wise, S.P. (1985). *Annu. Rev. Neurosci.* **8**, 1-19.

2

SUPPLEMENTARY MOTOR CORTEX AND SELF-INITIATED MOVEMENT

R.E. PASSINGHAM, Y.C. CHEN, AND D. THALER

Department of Experimental Psychology, University of Oxford, Oxford OX1 3UD, U.K.

Consider a dog lying on the floor. It comes when its master calls; but there are also occasions on which it gets up and comes of its own accord. In the first case there is a change in the environment; it hears the call. In the second case there is no change in the environment; instead there is a change in the animal itself. We can say that in the one instance the animal reacts to an external event, and that in the other its action is self-initiated.

It has been suggested that the supplementary motor cortex (SMA) plays a role in self-initiated movement (*1*). Three studies have compared the activity of cells in the SMA when monkeys make movements that are either self-paced or externally cued. Okano and Tanji (*7*) and Thaler *et al.* (*19*) compared movements made to a sound or to a time cue. Romo and Schultz (*12*) compared conditions when the animal reached for food either in its own time or when the door to the food box opened.

There are two findings. First, the studies agree that many cells are active in both conditions, that is, whether the animal is given an external signal or not. Second, there are indications that the time at which the cells become active differs on the two sorts of task. Okano and Tanji (*7*) divided cells into "long lead" cells that alter their discharge more than 480 msec before movement and "short lead" cells that do so less than 480 msec before movement; they found that in the SMA there are proportionately more long lead cells in the unsignalled than in the signalled condition. Thaler *et al.* (*19*) also compared the latencies for 30 cells tested on the two conditions; on the unsignalled task 33 percent of cells fired more than 230 msec before the earliest EMG, and on the signalled task the proportion was 18 percent. Romo and Schultz (*12*) report for the SMA that 25 percent of cells fire early on the self-initiated task.

However, there is less agreement on the degree to which the SMA is specialized for the production of self-initiated actions. Romo and Schultz (*12*) report that 32 percent of cells in the premotor cortex also respond early on the self-initiated task. But Okano and Tanji (*7*) compared the proportion of long lead cells recorded on the self-paced as opposed to the signalled task; there were proportionately more such cells in the SMA than in the premotor cortex.

There is a more critical test. If the SMA plays a crucial role in self-initiated movement two predictions follow. 1) Removal of the SMA should interfere with the production of such movements. 2) Removal of the premotor cortex should have no such effect. We report here on the results of such a test.

I. SELF-INITIATED ACTIONS

We have trained monkeys to perform a simple movement. (The term "movement" will usually be used even though the term "action" is strictly the more correct). The monkeys sit in a cage, and whenever they want a peanut they have simply to reach through the bars and raise an arm. If their hand cuts an invisible infrared beam a peanut is automatically delivered to a foodwell at the bottom of the cage. There is no visible target and there is no change in their environment to tell the animals when to raise their arm.

In our initial experiments we trained monkeys in the dark so as to be quite sure that there were no visible cues. We compared the four sessions after surgery with the four sessions immediately preceding surgery. Each session consisted of 65 trials.

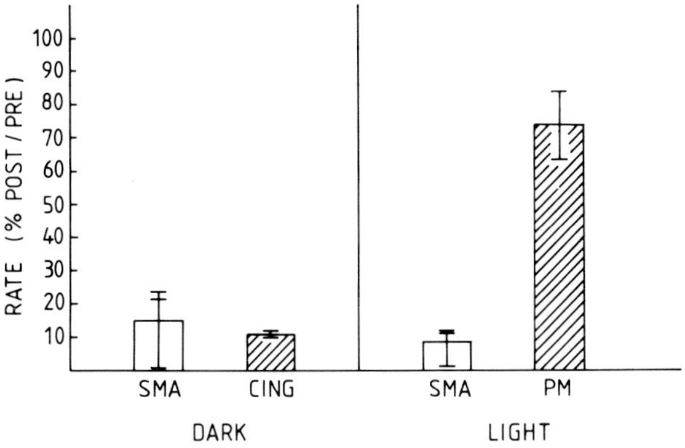

Fig. 1. Actions per minute on the self-initiated version of arm-raise task. The ordinate gives the percentage post-operative rate compared with the preoperative rate. The mean for the group is given by the histogram and the scores for each animal by the bars. SMA = supplementary motor cortex, CING = cingulate, PM = premotor. Dark = tested in the dark, Light = tested in the light. Data for SMA from Thaler (*17*), and for cingulate from Stern (*13*).

In three monkeys we removed the SMA bilaterally, including the upper bank of the cingulate sulcus. These animals were studied by Thaler (*17*), and he gives illustrations of the lesions. In two other monkeys we removed the lower bank of the cingulate sulcus, together with the rest of the anterior cingulate cortex, area 24. Stimulation of the lower bank of the cingulate sulcus can evoke movements (*6*); and there are independent projections to the motor cortex from this area (*16*). The cingulate operations were performed by D. Gaffan; they are illustrated in Stern (*13*).

Figure 1 shows the performance of the animals after surgery compared with their performance immediately before surgery. The monkeys with SMA lesions made few successful movements. The monkeys with cingulate lesions studied by Stern (*13*) were just as impaired.

In later experiments Thaler (*17*) taught other monkeys to raise their arm as before, but tested them in the light. They could see their arms as they reached, but there was no visible target. Figure 1 shows that under these conditions the monkeys with SMA lesions were as impaired as the monkeys that had been tested in the dark.

We also compared their performance with that of two monkeys

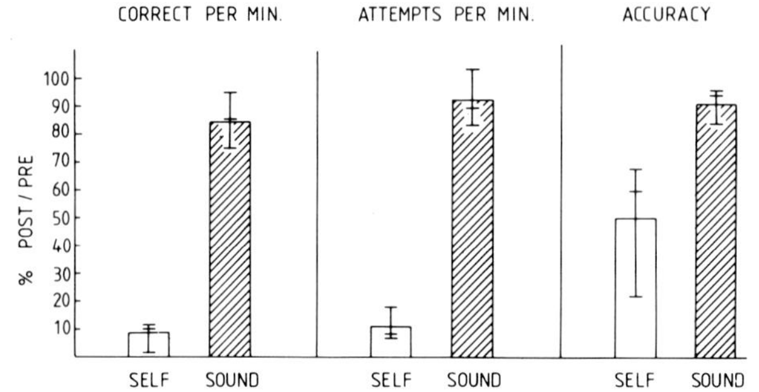

Fig. 2. Comparison of monkeys with SMA lesions and PM lesions on self-initiated version of arm-raise task. Ordinate and abbreviations as for Fig. 1. See text for definition of attempts and accuracy.

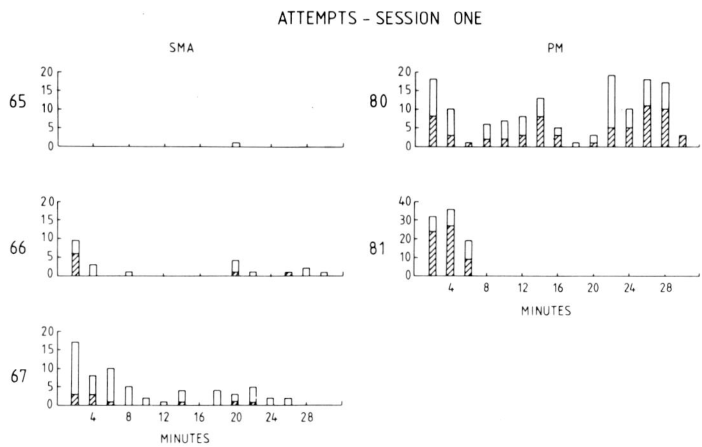

Fig. 3. Attempts and accuracy of attempts for the first post-operative session on the self-initiated arm-raise task. The attempts are shown by the clear histograms, and the successful attempts by the filled section of the histograms. The number of each animal is given to the left of each row. The session lasts up to 30 min.

with bilateral removal of the lateral premotor cortex. These lesions were like those reported by Passingham (*10*) except that the tissue above the level of the precentral sulcus was deliberately spared so as to minimize overlap with the SMA. These animals were studied by Chen (to be published). The animals raised their arms at a slightly slower rate than before surgery; but their performance was still greatly superior to that of the monkeys with SMA lesions (Fig. 1).

The difference between the monkeys with SMA lesions and premotor lesions is highlighted by the analysis shown in Fig. 2. We analyzed videotape of the animals' performance in the four sessions before and the four sessions after surgery. We noted the attempts the animals made, that is, the occasions on which they reached out of the cage; and we also noted the success of the attempts, that is, the occasions on which the animals interrupted the beam. The monkeys with premotor lesions made many more attempts, and were more accurate in their attempts, than the monkeys with SMA lesions (Fig. 2).

Figure 3 clearly shows the dramatic difference between the monkeys with SMA lesions and premotor lesions. The figure plots the attempts made by each animal in their first post-operative sessions, and also shows which attempts were accurate. One monkey with an SMA lesion made only one attempt; the other two made more attempts, but with little success. The animals with premotor lesions made many more attempts from the outset.

II. REACTIONS TO EXTERNAL EVENTS

If the SMA is concerned primarily with self-initiated movements monkeys with lesions in the SMA should have little trouble in reacting to external events. We trained three monkeys to raise their arm as before, but with the constraint that a peanut could be obtained only if the animal raised its arm within 2 sec after a tone sounded. If the animal raised its arm at other times the lights went out for 2 sec and no peanut arrived. This study was conducted by Chen (to be published).

Again, we removed the SMA bilaterally in three monkeys, and compared their performance in the first four post-operative sessions with that for the last four pre-operative sessions. The results are shown in Fig. 4 which also repeats the data from Fig. 2 for the SMA monkeys performing self-initiated movements. On the version with the sound cue the monkeys were almost as successful as they had been before surgery. They made many attempts and the majority of their attempts were accurate.

Several things are clear from these results. First, monkeys with

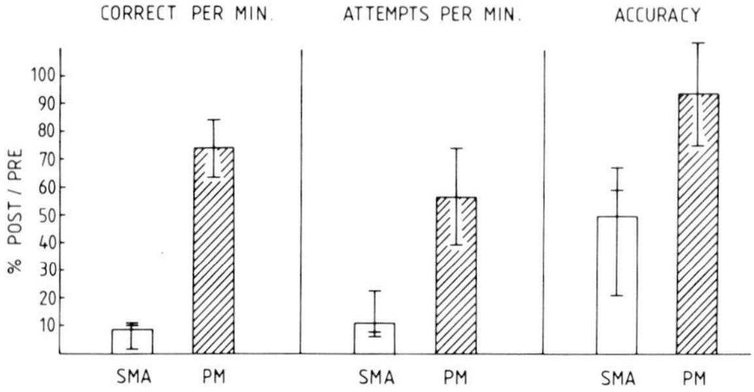

Fig. 4. Performance of monkeys with SMA lessions on self-initiated version of arm-raise task (self) and the version with a sound signal (sound). Ordinate and abbreviations as for Fig. 2.

SMA lesions are motivated to perform to obtain food; their failure to make many attempts on the self-initiated version does not mean that they will no longer work for food. Second, monkeys with SMA lesions can execute the required action; they are not impaired on the self-initiated version because they have some difficulty in raising their arm. Finally, the monkeys with SMA lesions can guide their hand to the correct position in space. Passingham (*9*) suggested that they might have difficulty in locating a target position as defined by propioceptive input. The present results show that this is not the case, since they can reach accurately if a sound cue is provided, even though they must still locate the same target position.

III. CHOICE BETWEEN TWO MOVEMENTS

Two explanations remain to explain the effect of adding the sound cue. The first is that the sound tells the animal *when* it can make a movement. The second explanation is that the sound reminds the animal *what* movement to make. We can distinguish these views by saying that the sound acts on the one hand as a trigger and on the other as an instruction (*18*). These two contributions can be distinguished by devising a task in which an external cue serves as a trigger but does not serve to remind the animal of the correct response.

This can be arranged by teaching the animal not one but two actions. We have taught monkeys to move a handle. The handle could either be pulled or it could be turned to the left; the apparatus is illustrated in Passingham (*10*). On each trial the monkey must choose which movement to perform. A simple rule specifies which movement is correct: on any day only one of the two actions will be correct, but if on one day the animal reaches a criterion level of 90% correct trials the conditions reverse and on the next day the other movement is defined as correct. Thus the animal learns a series of reversals.

This motor reversal task differs in one important respect from the task used for a recording study by Kurata and Wise (*3*). They reported little difference between the activity of cells in the SMA and premotor cortex when monkeys performed a spatial reversal task. This task required the animal to reverse between pressing a touchpad on the left or right, that is, between two locations. The motor reversal task differs in that it requires the animal to change between pulling and turning a handle, that is, between two movements. In the first case the monkey has only to recall the correct location (left or right) and then reach to a visuospatial target; in the second case the monkey has to recall which movement to make (pull or turn) as specified by propioceptive targets.

On the motor reversal task each trial starts with a screen being raised to allow the animal access to the handle. This event serves as an external trigger, telling the animal *when* it can respond. The crucial element in the design is that this cue does not tell the animal *what* action to take. The apparatus looks identical from trial to trial and there is no change in the environment to remind the animal how to succeed in winning food. In other words, while there is an external trigger there is no external event to act as an instruction.

We have taught this task after surgery to three groups of monkeys: Thaler (*17*) trained monkeys with bilateral SMA lesions; Chen (to be published) trained monkeys with bilateral premotor lesions; and three control monkeys were trained by Stern (*13*) and Thaler (*17*). The results are given in Fig. 5. The monkeys with premotor lesions performed as well as the control animals. Of the monkeys with SMA lesions two were very impaired, taking very many trials to master five reversals. The third animal also took more trials than the control animals, but was less impaired. Unfortunately, the training of this animal was disrupted because the monkey was

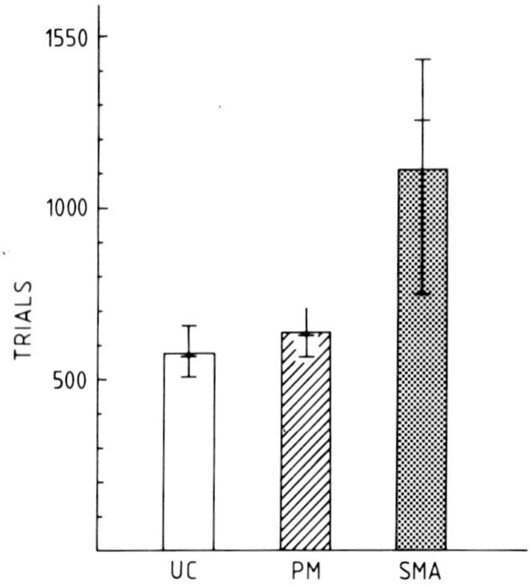

Fig. 5. Trials to learn 5 reversals on motor reversal task. Abbreviations as for other figures.

quarantined due to illness in the colony; after one reversal further training had to be postponed until 2 months later.

These data confirm conclusions from the earlier study. The monkeys with SMA lesions are motivated to perform to obtain food. Furthermore, they can execute the relevant movement; it was not that they could not pull or turn the handle, but that they pulled when they should have turned and *vice versa.*

These data resolve the issue of why monkeys with SMA lesions can perform the arm-raise task with a sound cue. The cue does not help because it serves as a trigger to tell them *when* to respond; on the reversal task the monkeys are impaired even though there is an external trigger to serve this function. The sound cue helps because it serves as an instruction to remind the animals *what* to do.

It follows that the animals should be able to pull or turn a handle correctly if provided with an external cue to tell them which to do. We have previously described such a task. The cue is shown on a TV monitor; the rule is that if a blue patch is shown the animal should pull the handle, but that if a red one is shown the animal should turn the handle. This visual conditional task was taught by P.D. Nixon to three monkeys, and we then removed the SMA bilaterally. After surgery the monkeys relearned the task very quickly

(*9*). Clearly, their problem with the motor reversal task is not that they perseverate and are unable to pull or turn the handle flexibly. Their problem is that there is no external cue and they have problems in knowing on any trial which movement to make.

IV. DISCUSSION

When the movements are self-initiated monkeys with SMA lesions do little in the first few sessions. It would be usual to say that they no longer "initiate" actions. However, this description can be misleading, as it may be taken to suggest either that the animals lack the motivation to act or that they are unable, in some way, to get started. Yet it is clear that neither explanation is correct, since the animals produce many actions if there is a sound cue.

It is more profitable to discuss the matter in terms of a problem with "retrieval". When a person tries to find a word some search must take place to locate the word in memory and retrieve it (*14*). A word processor does the same when it searches for a file or conducts a spelling check. The production of movements must involve a similar process. If movements are learned then some search must be made for the *appropriate* movement given the present context. Passingham (*11*) has argued elsewhere that the retrieval of the appropriate movement depends on the premotor strip, including the SMA.

It is a property of such retrieval mechanisms that an item may be retrieved under one condition and not under another (*20*). A person fails to think of a name but can do so when prompted, for example by being given the first letter of the name. One way in which an external prompt can aid recall is by specifying the point at which the search should start.

The suggestion is that on the arm raise task the monkeys with SMA lesions fail to make attempts because they are unable to retrieve the appropriate movement without a reminder. The analogy is with aphasic patients who are mute, not because they make no effort to speak but because the appropriate words do not come to mind. It is an intriguing fact that large infarcts of the medial frontal cortex, including the SMA and cingulate gyrus, can cause patients to be mute; yet these same patients can sometimes speak if prompted by questions (*2*, *4*). Like the monkeys described here, they are better at reacting than they are at acting of their own accord.

A related phenomenon occurs in Parkinson's disease. Patients may be akinetic when left to move on their own, and yet able to move when prompted by external cues. Thus the patient may be able to catch a ball, but then be unable to throw it back. This phenomenon is know as "paradoxical kinesis" (*5*). There are two views. 1) The usual view has been that the patient needs a stimulus to motivate him. When a ball comes towards him the patient is surprised and is thus stirred into action; when the patient must throw there is no boost to the patient's motivation. 2) An alternative view is that the patient needs a reminder as to what to do. When the ball comes towards him there is a change in the environment, and the patient reacts to this event; when the patient must throw there is no change in the environment, and the patient must initiate the action himself. It is of interest that there is a report that a tumour in the SMA can produce Parkinsonian symptoms (*15*).

The same distinction is evident in studies of gross electrical potentials in human subjects. It is possible to record the Bereitschaft-potential (BP) over the vertex when a person decides upon an action. Papa *et al.* (*8*) asked subjects in one condition to extend the right wrist at their own pace, and in another to either extend the right wrist or supinate the left in any order that they chose. In both conditions the BP could be recorded. However, the BP could not be detected if an external signal told them either when to make the movement or which of the two movements to make.

Both in monkeys and in human subjects there seems to be a crucial distinction between those actions that are taken as a result of a change in the environment and those actions that are decided by the subject in the absence of such a change. The dictionary allows the use of the word "voluntary" for those actions that are taken without external prompting; but it seems odd to refer to reactions as "involuntary". In ordinary language, when the dog answers the call its behaviour is no less voluntary than when it gets up of its own accord. Whatever word is used the distinction appears to be a fundamental one in terms of the brain mechanisms involved.

SUMMARY

Animals perform some acts of their own accord and some in response to external events. It is argued that the premotor areas in general are concerned with the retrieval of the appropriate movements, and that the SMA in particular is concerned with the retrieval of self-initiated movements. Evidence is cited from experiments on monkeys with lesions in the SMA or premotor cortex.

Monkeys were trained to reach out into midair, so interrupting an invisible infrared beam which operates the peanut dispenser. Monkeys with SMA lesions were poor at making such movements under self-paced conditions; but monkeys with premotor lesions made more attempts and were more accurate in their attempts.

Monkeys with SMA lesions were much better if a sound was provided to remind them what to do. It is argued that external cues help, not because they tell the animal *when* to act, but because they tell them *what* to do. Monkeys with SMA lesions were poor on a motor reversal task, even though an external cue told them when to act. On this task there is no external cue to tell them which movement to make.

REFERENCES

1 Eccles, J.C. (1982). *Arch. Psychiatr. Nervenkr.* **231**, 423-441.
2 Jonas, S. (1987). In *The Frontal Lobes Revisited*, ed. Perecman, E., pp. 241-250. New York: IRBN Press.
3 Kurata, K. and Wise, S.P. (1988). *Exp. Brain Res.* **72**, 237-248.
4 Laplane, D., Tailarach, J., Meininger, V., Bancaud, J., and Orgogozo, J.M. (1977), *J. Neurol. Sci.* **34**, 301-314.
5 Marsden, C.D., Parkes, J.D., and Quinn, N. (1982). In *Movement Disorders*, ed. Marsden, C.D. and Fahn, S., pp. 96-122. London: Butterworth.
6 Mitz, A.R. and Wise, S.P. (1987). *J. Neurosci.* **9**, 1010-1021.
7 Okano, K. and Tanji, J. (1987). *Exp. Brain Res.* **66**, 155-166.
8 Papa, S.M., Artieda, J., and Obeso, J.A. Abstract for Meeting on Neural Mechanisms in Disorders of Movement, 1988, Manchester.
9 Passingham, R.E. (1987). In *Motor Areas of the Cerebral Cortex*, ed. Porter, R., pp. 151-161. Chichester: John Wiley & Sons.
10 Passingham, R.E. (1988). *Exp. Brain Res.* **70**, 590-596.

11 Passingham, R.E. *Brain Beh. Evol.*, in press.
12 Romo, R. and Schultz, W. (1987). *Exp. Brain Res.* **67**, 656–662.
13 Stern, C.E. (1987). *Functions of the Ventral Striatum*, Ph.D. Thesis, Oxford University, unpublished.
14 Sternberg, S. (1975). *Quart. J. Exp. Psychol.* **27**, 1–32.
15 Straube, A. and Sigel, K. (1988). *J. Neurol. Neurosurg. Psychiatr.* **51**, 730–731.
16 Strick, P. (1985). *Beh. Brain Res.* **18**, 107–124.
17 Thaler, D.E. (1988). *Supplementary Motor Cortex and the Control of Action*, Ph.D. Thesis, Oxford University, unpublished.
18 Thaler, D.E. and Passingham, R.E. (1989) In *Neural Mechanisms in Disorders of Movement*, ed. Crossman, A.R. and Sambrook, M.A., pp. 175–182. London: Libbey.
19 Thaler, D.E., Rolls, E.T., and Passingham, R.E. *Neurosci. Lett.* **93**, 264–269.
20 Tulving, E. (1983). *Elements of Episodic Memory*. Oxford: Oxford University Press.

3

FRONTAL CORTEX ACTIVITY AND MOTOR SET

STEVEN P. WISE

Laboratory of Neurophysiology, National Institute of Mental Health, Poolesville, Maryland 20837, U.S.A.

This discussion will address two topics and their conjunction: the concept of *behavioral set* and neuronal activity during *instructed delay periods.* Behavioral set is the process of preparing for some event that will take place in the future. Instructed delay periods are times when an experimental subject withholds a specific act, and neuronal activity during that period has been termed *delay-period activity.* Two propositions will be central to the present discussion. One is that behavioral set can be understood as a group of related processes, a set in a different sense of the term. The other is that many cortical fields (and some subcortical structures) exhibit delay-period activity. These propositions raise the possibility that delay-period activity in the various cortical fields that evince it underlies a distinct set-related process in each field.

I. BEHAVIORAL SET

Set has been defined as "a state of readiness to receive a stimulus that has not yet arrived or a state of readiness to make a movement" (*14, 73*). Another term that has been used in this context is *preparation,* meaning the preparation for events that have not yet occurred or actions that are to be performed in the future. The concepts are not quite identical, set (preparedness) is the state that preparation establishes, but there is sufficient similarity that they can be used interchangeably for most purposes.

Despite the reification that might be implicit in the use of a single term, set has not been thought of as an indivisible process. A distinction has been repeatedly made, for example, between sensory and motor aspects of set. A stage (*57*) or process (*44*) of response preparation, distinct from preparation to receive sensory information, is inherent in most models of reaction-time behavior. Sensory set is most commonly called selective attention; motor set has often been termed intention. Whereas it might appear unattractive, at first glance, to consider attention and intention together, as Hebb (*29*) argued, "attention is selectivity in what is responded to, or sensory selectivity; [intentional] set is a selectivity of response, motor rather than sensory". More recently, other investigators have also remarked upon the close relationship of attention and motor set, establishing a link of concepts if not of processes. It has often been noted that, as one cannot make a limb movement in several directions at once, so it appears to be impossible to direct attention to several parts of space or to several objects at once. Indeed, the concepts of motor set and attention are sufficiently similar that the term "motor attention" has been proposed for motor aspects of set (*25*). Thus, in this view, the hierarchically superior concept of attention can be subdivided into sensory and motor aspects. In an alternative view (*14*) the hierarchically superior concept of set can be subdivided into sensory (attentional) aspects and motor (intentional) aspects.

II. FRONTAL CORTEX ACTIVITY

1. *Neurophysiological Nomenclature*

Numerous reports show that cells in the frontal cortex have at least four patterns of discharge modulation during visuomotor tasks. Unfortunately, the nomenclature employed in these reports is virtually identical to their number and tends, therefore, to vary for studies involving slightly different tasks or cortical fields. Typically, however, the tasks that have been used involve: 1) an *intertrial interval* in which the monkey awaits a cue, 2) an *instruction stimulus*, informing the animal about the movement to be executed or the target of that movement, 3) an *instructed delay period* during which the monkey must withhold the behavior, 4) a *trigger stimulus*, that signals the monkey to initiate the movement, and 5) the behavior itself, leading to reward if correctly executed. *Precue activity*, precedes the instruction stimulus if it occurs at a relatively predictable time (*43, 63*). This pattern of activity has also been termed anticipatory (*10, 43*) or attention-related (*6*). *Postcue activity*, appears to be a phasic and time-locked response to the sensory instruction stimulus and has also been termed signal-related (*68*), visual (*10, 24*) or phasic (*54*). *Delay-period activity**, which persists from soon after the instruction stimulus until approximately the beginning of movement has also been termed set-related (*68*), preparatory (*33, 51*), visuomotor (*10, 24*), or tonic (*54*). And, *premovement activity*, which precedes and is time-locked with movement onset (*68, 69, 72*), has been variously termed movement-related or motor activity. Combinations of these patterns are commonly observed in individual neurons (see, *e.g.*, refs. *18, 51,* and *72*, for recent descriptions of this phenomenon).

2. *Delay-period Activity*

Delay-period activity was first described in the prefrontal (*16, 17, 36*) and primary motor cortex (*15*), observations that have been repeated many times (*18, 34, 35, 47, 48, 59, 62, 64, 66, 69*). The observation of delay-period activity has since been extended to the supplementary motor cortex (*37, 60, 61*), premotor cortex (*21, 51, 68*), frontal eye field (*10*), and the cingulate cortex (*49*) (see Fig. 1). No doubt, other frontal fields will soon be added to the list, especially as those fields become better defined. Additionally, delay-period activity has been observed in structures that provide inputs to the frontal cortex, such as the cerebellum (*58, 62*) and both areas 5 and 7 of the posterior parietal cotex (*11, 22, 23*). At least one target of frontal corticofugal projections, the putamen (*1*) shows delay-period activity, as does the hippocampal formation (*67*), which is, according to some experts,

*Delay-period activity was also termed anticipatory discharge by Evarts and Tanji (*15, 59*).

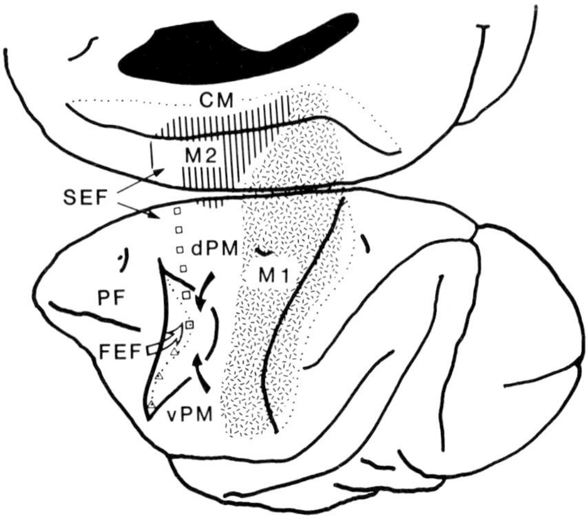

Fig. 1. Diagram of the left hemisphere of a macaque monkey, with the medial aspect of the hemisphere reflected at the top. The best-defined areas of the frontal cortex are approximately located. CM, cingulate motor field(s); dPM, dorsal premotor cortex; FEF, frontal eye field; M1, primary motor cortex; M2, supplementary motor cortex; PF, prefrontal cortex; SEF, supplementary eye field; vPM, ventral premotor cortex.

closely associated with the frontal cortex and the control of motor behavior (*27, 53*).

The hypothesis that delay-period activity in the premotor cortex reflects the preparation for specific motor actions has been the subject of numerous tests, which have yielded results consistent with that hypothesis (*38, 39, 70*). And although delay-period activity in other frontal cortical fields has not been studied in the same manner, it appears likely that at least some of it also reflects aspects of motor preparation. For example, the effect of cortical damage to the supplementary motor cortex (and its vicinity) has been linked to deficits in intention (*65*), as contrasted with attention, and it seems likely that the delay period activity observed there may play a role in that function.

III. ASPECTS OF MOTOR SET

There appear to be several aspects of motor set. Some of these, namely motor programming (*i.e.*, the specification of the time and force parameters for a movement), retrieval of motor programs, reaction time and reflex modulation, and suppression of what might be termed "direct action" circuits, will be discussed below in the context of neurophysiological data. Other aspects will be neglected here, but this should not be taken to imply that those facets of set are any less important in the adaptive preparation for action. For example, the regulation of posture, especially of the proximal and axial musculature for the purpose of providing a stable base for distal limb action (and for other purposes) is an essential part of motor preparation (*31*, *32*). Furthermore, autonomic reactions to the environment also contribute to the preparation for action at a future time. In chimpanzees, faster reaction times are correlated with higher heart rate, and target detection (during a period of expectancy) is usually followed by cardiac acceleration (*7*). In humans, after an instruction that informs a subject about the movement that is to be made, there is a triphasic alteration in heart rate, an early decrease followed by an increase and a subsequent decrease, which precedes a cue that triggers the movement (*12*). Finally, cognitive aspects of behavioral set, perhaps its most important facet, will also be ignored here. This, despite the recognition that the ability to predict events represents one of the highest of brain functions. Indeed, the teleonomic function of the learning and memory mechanisms of the vertebrate brain can be viewed as serving the single purpose of preparation for future action.

1. Reaction-time Modulation

The functional significance of long-latency, transcortical stretch reflexes, indeed their very existence, has been controversial. However, it is unquestioned that the magnitude of EMG modulations occurring at "reflex" latencies ($<<100$ msec) can be much affected by the instructions that are given to the subject (*8*, *9*, *14*, *52*). In one set of studies, the magnitude of long-latency reflexes was measured during different parts of an instructed delay period. It was found that when the subjects needed to respond as rapidly as possible, that an instruction to flex the wrist led to an increase stretch response from the flexor muscles of the wrist. Following an instruction that the soon-to-be-triggered movement was an extension, the long-latency response in the flexor muscles decreased, a pattern of response that is precisely what would be needed for expediting reactions. For example, by decreasing the stiffness of the wrist flexors while they are being passively lengthened, the viscoelastic resistance (or mechanical impedance) of the limb would be reduced and the response could, in principle, occur faster. It has been argued that the effects observed by Bonnet (*8*) and Bonnet and Requin (*9*) may have been due to co-contraction of flexors and extensors during the delay period (*52*), but that would appear to account only for increases where observed, but not the observed decreases in response amplitude.

There is no direct evidence that cortical delay-period activity underlies the modulation of response amplitude at these latencies. However, Hummelsheim *et al.* (*30*) have reported that electrical stimulation of the supplementary motor area (M2) leads to smaller and slower responses to kinesthetic stimuli among primary motor cortex (M1) neurons. Thus, one multipart hypothesis is that delay-period neurons in M2 project to M1 (hypothesis 1) and inhibit its responses (hypothesis 2) to stretch-receptor inputs (hypothesis 3). Such a mechanism could underlie the regulation of long-latency reflexes observed by Bonnett (*8*). This view is also consistent with the observations that damage to M2 "releases" grasping reflexes (*56*).

However, areas other than M2 may also play a role in regulation of long-latency stretch (or other) responses. Some investigators have argued that if delay-period activity plays a role in expediting reactions, the magnitude of neuronal modulation should correlate with reaction time. Although this is not a necessary prediction of the hypothesis in question, it represents a part of one possible mechanism through which delay-period activity could affect reaction time. Requin and his colleagues (*41, 51*) have been able to document the activity of delay-period neurons in both premotor cortex (PM) and primary motor cortex (M1) that have this property: the magnitude of delay-period activity inversely correlates with reaction time.

Although it remains to be established whether delay-period neurons of this or any other type are corticofugal cells, corticocortical cells, or both, it is plausible that these cells play some role in expediting reactions through either pathway. Among its corticocortical projections, PM has long been known to project to both M2 and

M1, and either of these projections might be important in the regulation of long-latency stretch responses. Thus, one aspect of motor set in which delay-period activity may be involved is the expedition of reactions on the basis of expectation or prior instruction, possibly through a mechanism that involves the modulation of long-latency responses to kinesthetic stimuli and possibly involving cell activity that decreases reaction time in proportion to the magnitude of its delay-period activity.

2. Suppression of Direct Action Circuits

Encephalization, *i.e.*, the progressive arrogation of behavioral control by telencephalic, as opposed to more caudal, structures is a venerable concept in neurology. In this view, one duty in the cortical control of movement is to suppress "lower", direct action circuits. Evidence in favor of this idea comes from clinical studies, which have specifically implicated the frontal lobes in this sort of function. It has been found that patients with damage to the frontal cortex have difficulty suppressing saccades to a visual target that appears in peripheral vision. Importantly, these "unwanted" saccades are of very short latency compared to "voluntary" eye movements (*28*). Guitton and his colleagues concluded:

> . . . . the frontal lobes, particularly the dorsolateral region which contains the (frontal eye field) and possibly the supplementary motor area contribute to the generation of complex saccadic eye-movement behaviour. More specifically, they appear to aid in *suppressing* unwanted reflex-like oculomotor activity and in *triggering* the appropriate volitional movements when the goal for the movement is known but not yet visible (ref. *28*, italics original).

In the skeletomotor system, a perhaps not dissimilar phenomenon is seen in the alien hand syndrome (*26*), thought to be caused by medial frontal damage. In that syndrome, involuntary, but seemingly purposive (and, in any event, well organized) forelimb movements appear to be out of the control of the patient. It is not too fanciful to link these two phenomena under the general heading of stimulus-linked behavior unfettered by normal suppressive influences. Indeed, one recent model of working memory has posited the existence of a central executive that functions, in part, to suppress relatively automatic behaviors (*4*). And, as with the production of unwanted saccades, the loss of executive function has been linked to frontal lobe damage (*5*).

This general idea is supported by studies in nonhuman animals. For example, eye movements to visual targets occur with a bimodal temporal distribution. Ablation of the superior colliculus of monkeys causes the shortest mode (about 80 msec) to disappear; ablation of the frontal eye field does not (*55*). Thus, it appears likely that the fastest oculomotor reactions, perhaps those made by the frontal-lobe-damaged patients described by Guitton *et al.* (*28*), are mediated *via* brainstem circuits. Moll and Kuypers (*46*) also proposed a specific, suppressive role for PM and M2 based on the effects of cortical ablations. They found that monkeys with lesions to those two areas could not learn to reach around a transparent barrier in order to obtain a food reward. Instead, the monkey perseverated in reaching directly toward the food, thereby encountering the barrier and failing to obtain rewards. Intact monkeys, of course, have no difficulty learning the complex movement trajectories necessary to obtain the reward. Moll and Kuypers (*46*) interpreted the lesioned animals inabilities to a lack of suppression of the direct reaching movement.

More recently, this view of frontal lobe function has received further support from cortical stimulation studies, at least for PM of humans. Lüders *et al.* (*42*) have stimulated the surface of the cortex in awake patients and found that stimulation immediately rostral to M1 causes a rapid suppression of ongoing movements in a roughly topographic pattern, with lateral PM stimulation stopping orofacial movements and more medial stimulation disrupting arm movements.

Some properties of delay-period activity in PM supports the idea that frontal areas play a role in suppression of movements. First, some delay-period neurons lack movement-related activity and are active only when an animal suppresses a previously instructed movement (*72*). Other delay-period neurons, such as that illustrated in Fig. 2 have more complicated patterns of activity. This cell discharges significantly after the trigger stimulus, except in the bottom four trials (*71*). In those four trials, the trigger stimulus was delayed and activity

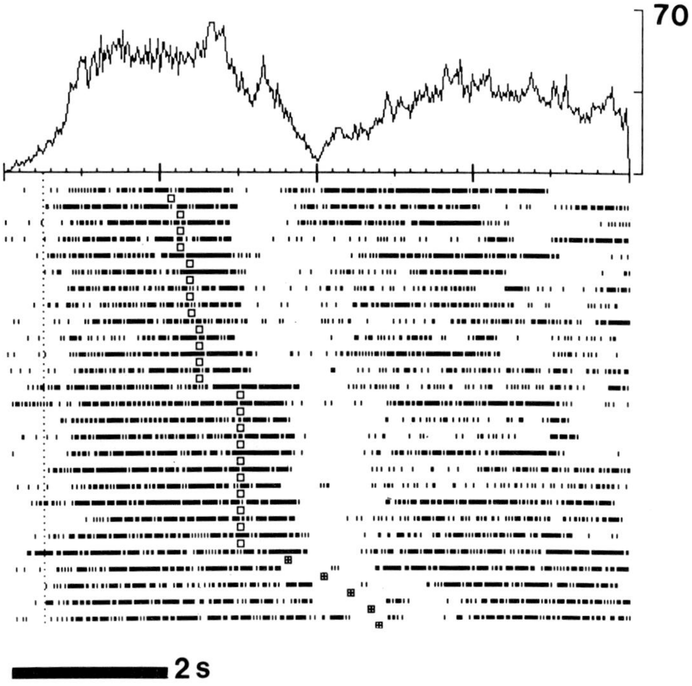

Fig. 2. Activity of one PM neuron. The average reciprocal interval plot is shown at the top, the raster of neuronal activity is shown at the bottom. The vertical dotted line shows the time, during each trial, when a visuospatial instruction stimulus was presented to the monkey. The square beneath the raster lines shows the time when a trigger stimulus was presented, and the squares with crosses inside (bottom four trials) indicate trials in which the monkey fails to withhold movement for the required period. In those bottom four trials the onset of movement occurred at the time indicated by the square and it can be observed that the cell ceases discharging long before such failures to suppress the previously instructed movement.

ceases long before any trigger stimulus is delivered (*71*). The cessation of activity correlates well with the failure to continue withholding the instructed movement, just as one would predict of a circuit playing a suppressive role in motor control. Kurata and Tanji (*37*) have made similar arguments regarding delay-period activity in M2. Neither these nor any other delay-period neurons, at least in PM, appear to reflect, in their magnitude of activity, any parameter of movement (*e.g.*, velocity, force, or acceleration) with the possible exception of reaction time (noted above) and the certain exception of direction (*18, 51, 62, 68, 69*). Such a lack of relationship with motor parameters (except, perhaps, movement direction) would be expected of a switching mechanism: it is either on or off for a given movement.

Although the neuronal evidence cited above needs to be bolstered by direct experimentation, it seems plausible that delay-period activity may play a role in suppressing the expression of direct, relatively automatic, and presumably brainstem-mediated limb projection movements. The pathways through which this suppression could be effected are not known, but it is worth noting that one of the major, if not the major, efferent projections of PM is to the medullary magnocellular reticular formation (*40*). That brainstem target has long been held to be the source inhibitory reticulospinal influences (*2, 3, 13*).

3. Retrieval of Movements from Memory

Passingham (*50*) has recently proposed that an aspect of motor preparation in which the premotor cortex participates is the retrieval of the movement to be executed on the basis of stimulus context. This hypothesis is consistent with the neurophysiological findings of Sasaki and his colleagues, who have studied slow-wave activity during the learning of simple visually triggered movements and concluded that the premotor cortex participates in a kind of motor learning (*19, 20*). In order to further and more explicitly test this hypothesis, Andrew Mitz, Moshe Godschalk, and I designed an experiment aimed at examining neuronal activity while a monkey acquired a visuomotor association. The details of the experimental design and results will be reported at a later date, but preliminary results from the experiment indicate that PM cells change their activity dramatically while the monkey learns a new (and arbitrary) visuomotor association. This finding implies that some PM neurons mediate the selection and/or execution movement on the basis of learned sensorimotor association and that parallel circuits (in PM or elsewhere) mediate the selection of movements on other bases, operative when the monkey must "guess" the appropriate response to a novel stimulus.

IV. CONCLUSION

Delay-period activity is widely distributed in the frontal cortex, as well as in structures that provide its inputs to and receive its outputs. There is evidence (not presented here) that delay-period activity in PM reflects some aspect of the preparation for action, *i.e.*, behavioral set. It seems likely that delay-period activity elsewhere does too. Set is considered here, not as a monolithic, indivisible function or process, but rather as a set of related functions. Just as behavioral set has its sensory (attentional) and its motor (intentional) aspects, so, too, motor set has several facets. Three of these facets, none exclusive of the others, were discussed in the context of delay-period activity that has been observed in the primate frontal cortex. Although any conclusion must be provisional at this time, there appears to be evidence that, among the roles of the premotor cortex in the preparation for future action, it is involved in the retrieval of a movement to be made on the basis of an arbitrary stimulus context (*50*). M2, and perhaps the delay-period activity in that field, appears to play some role in the modulation of the primary motor cortex responses to kinesthetic stimuli. In so doing it may be part of a mechanism that expedites reactions to predictable stimuli. In addition to M2, PM and other cortical fields may also play a role in this process. And PM and M2 together, perhaps in association with other frontal fields, may suppress direct, subcortically mediated actions. Delay-period activity has the properties expected of a component of such a circuit. In conclusion, it may be speculated by calling up new motor programs, suppressing other, automatically executed actions, and expediting the response to an expected stimulus, delay-period activity underlies the ability for flexible, rapid action (*14*).

SUMMARY

The concept of behavioral set is discussed as a set of processes involved in establishing a multifaceted state of readiness for environmental events not yet occurring and movements not yet made. These processes include, but are not restricted to, retrieving a movement from memory, establishing a motor program, adjusting posture, suppressing "direct action" circuits, and adjusting autonomic tone. Delay-period activity, especially in the frontal cortex, may participate in the mechanisms of these and other preparatory processes.

REFERENCES

1 Alexander, G.E. (1987). *Exp. Brain Res.* **67**, 623–634.
2 Alstermark, B., Lundberg, A., and Sasaki, S. (1984a). *Exp. Brain Res.* **56**, 293–307.
3 Alstermark, B., Lundberg, A., and Sasaki, S. (1984b). *Exp. Brain Res.* **56**, 308–322.
4 Baddeley, A.D. (1986). *Working Memory.* London/New York: Oxford University Press.
5 Baddeley, A.D. and Wilson, B. (1988) *Brain and Cognition* **7**, 212–230.
6 Bakay Pragay, E., Mirsky, A.F., and Nakamura, R.K. (1987). *Exp. Neurol.* **96**, 481–500.
7 Berntson, G.G. and Boysen, S.T. (1987). *Psychobiology* **15**, 87–92.
8 Bonnet, M. (1983). *Brain Res.* **280**, 51–62.
9 Bonnet, M. and Requin, M. (1982). *J. Neurosci.* **2**, 90–96.
10 Bruce, C.J. and Goldberg, M.E. (1985). *J. Neurophysiol.* **53**, 603–635.
11 Crammond, D.J. and Kalaska, J.F. (1989). *Exp. Brain Res.*, in press.
12 Damen, E.J.P. and Brunia, C.H.M. (1987). *Psychophysiology* **24**, 700–713.
13 Engberg, I., Lundberg, A., and Ryall, R.W. (1968). *J. Physiol.* **194**, 201.
14 Evarts, E.V., Shinoda, Y., and Wise, S.P. (1984). *Neurophysiological Approaches to Higher Brain Function.* New York: John Wiley & Sons.
15 Evarts, E.V. and Tanji, J. (1974). *Brain Res.* **71**, 479–494.
16 Fuster, J.M. (1973). *J. Neurophysiol.* **36**, 61–78.
17 Fuster, J.M. and Alexander, G.E. (1971). *Science* **173**, 652–654.
18 Georgopoulos, A.P., Crutcher, M.D., and Schwartz, A.B. (1989). *Exp. Brain Res.* **75**, 183–194.
19 Gemba, H. and Sasaki, K. (1984). *Exp. Brain Res.* **55**, 26–32.
20 Gemba, H. and Sasaki, K. (1988). *Exp. Brain Res.* **70**, 43–49.
21 Godschalk, M. and Lemon, R.N. (1983). *Exp. Brain Res.* Suppl. **7**, 114–119.
22 Godschalk, M., Lemon, R.N., and Kuypers, H.G.J.M. (1984). *Experientia* **40**, 1297–1298.
23 Godschalk, M., Lemon, R.N., Kuypers, H.G.J.M., and Van Der Steen, J. (1985). *Behav. Brain Res.* **18**, 143–157.
24 Godschalk, M., Lemon, R.N., Nijs, H.G.T., and Kuypers, H.G.J.M. (1981). *Exp. Brain Res.* **44**, 113–116.
25 Goldberg, M.E. and Segraves, M.A. (1987). *Neuropsychologia* **25**, 107–118.
26 Goldberg, G., Mayer, N.H., and Toglia, J.U. (1981). *Arch Neurol.* **38**, 683–686.
27 Goldman-Rakic, P.S., Selemon, L.D., and Schwartz, M.L. (1984). *Neuroscience* **12**, 719–743.

28 Guitton, D., Buchtel, H.A., and Douglas, R.M. (1985). *Exp. Brain Res.* **58**, 455-472.
29 Hebb, D.O. (1972). In *Textbook of Psychology*, pp. 72-93. Philadelphia: Saunders.
30 Hummelsheim, M., Wiesendanger, M., and Bianchetti, M. (1986). *Neurosci. Lett.* **67**, 119-122.
31 Humphrey, D.R. (1979). In *Posture and Movement*, ed. Talbot, R.E. and Humphrey, D.R., pp. 51-112. New York: Raven Press.
32 Humphrey, D.R., Gold, R., and Reed, D.J. (1984). *J. Comp. Neurol.* **225**, 75-94.
33 Kubota, K. and Hamada, I. (1978). *J. Physiol.* **74**, 297-312.
34 Kubota, K. and Funahashi, S. (1982). *J. Neurophysiol.* **47**, 362-376.
35 Kubota, K., Iwamoto, T., and Suzuki, H. (1974). *J. Neurophysiol.* **36**, 1197-1212.
36 Kubota, K. and Niki, H. (1971). *J. Neurophysiol.* **34**, 337-347.
37 Kurata, K. and Tanji, J. (1985). *J. Neurophysiol.* **53**, 142-152.
38 Kurata, K. and Wise, S.P. (1988). *Exp. Brain Res.* **69**, 327-343.
39 Kurata, K. and Wise, S.P. (1988). *Exp. Brain Res.*, in press.
40 Kuypers, H.G.J.M. and Brinkman, J. (1970). *Brain Res.* **24**, 29-48.
41 Lecas, J.-C., Requin, J., Anger, C., and Vitton, N. (1986). *J. Neurophysiol.* **56**, 1680-1702.
42 Lüders, H., Lesser, R.P., Morris, H.H., Dinner, D.S., and Hahn, J. (1987). *Adv. Epileptol.* **16**, 229-231.
43 Mauritz, K.-H. and Wise, S.P. (1986). *Exp. Brain Res.* **61**, 229-244.
44 McClelland, J.L. (1979). *Psychol. Rev.* **86**, 287-330.
45 Meyer, D.E., Irwin, D.E., Osman, A.M., and Kounios, J. (1988). *Psychol. Rev.* **95**, 183-237.
46 Moll, L. and Kuypers, H.G.J.M. (1977). *Science* **198**, 317-319.
47 Niki, H. (1974). *Brain Res.* **68**, 185-196.
48 Niki, H. and Watanabe, M. (1976). *Brain Res.* **105**, 79-88.
49 Niki, H. and Watanabe, M. (1976). *Brain Res.* **110**, 381-386.
50 Passingham, R.E. (1988). *Exp. Brain Res.* **70**, 590-596.
51 Riehle, A. and Requin, J. (1988). *J. Neurophysiol.* **61**, 543-549.
52 Rothwell, J.C. (1987). In *Higher Brain Functions, Recent Explorations of the Brain's Emergent Properties*, ed. Wise, S.P., pp. 113-130. New York: John Wiley & Sons.
53 Rupniak, N.M. and Gaffan, D. (1987). *J. Neurosci.* **7**, 2332-2337.
54 Sawaguchi, T. (1987). *J. Neurophysiol.* **58**, 1080-1099.
55 Schiller, P.H., Sandell, H.J., and Maunsell, J.H.R. (1987). *J. Neurophysiol.* **57**, 1033-1049.
56 Smith, A.M., Bourbonnais, D., and Blanchette, G. (1981). *Brain Res.* **222**, 395-400.
57 Sternberg, S. (1969). In *Attention and Performance*, ed. Koster, W.G., pp. 276-315. Amsterdam: North Holland.
58 Strick, P.L. (1983). *J. Neurosci.* **3**, 2007-2020.
59 Tanji, J. and Evarts, E.V. (1976). *J. Neurophysiol.* **39**, 1062-1068.
60 Tanji, J. and Kurata, J. (1985). *J. Neurophysiol.* **43**, 60-68.

61 Tanji, J., Taniguchi, K., and Saga, T. (1980). *J. Neurophysiol.* **43**, 60–69.
62 Thach, W.T. (1978). *J. Neurophysiol.* **41**, 654–676.
63 Vaadia, E., Kurata, K., and Wise, S.P. (1988). *Somatosens. Mot. Res.* **6**, 207–230.
64 Vaadia, E., Benson, D.A., Hienz, R.D., and Goldstein, M.H. (1986). *J. Neurophysiol.* **56**, 934–952.
65 Valenstein, E., Watson, R.T., Van Den Abell, T., Carter, R., and Heilman, K.M. (1987). *Arch. Neurol.* **44**, 517–520.
66 Watanabe, M. (1981). *Brain Res.* **225**, 51–65.
67 Watanabe, M. and Niki, H. (1985). *Brain Res.* **325**, 242–254.
68 Weinrich, M. and Wise, S.P. (1982). *J. Neurosci.* **2**, 1329–1345.
69 Weinrich, M., Wise, S.P., and Mauritz, K.-H. (1984). *Brain* **107**, 385–414.
70 Wise, S.P. (1985). *Behav. Brain Res.* **18**, 79–88.
71 Wise, S.P. and Kurata, K. (1989). *Somatosens. Mot. Res.*, in press.
72 Wise, S.P., Weinrich, M., and Mauritz, K.-H. (1986). *Prog. Brain Res.* **64**, 117–131.
72 Woodworth, R.S. (1958). *Dynamics of Behavior.* New York: Holt, Rinehart and Winston.

4

MOTOR PROGRAMMING IN THE PREMOTOR CORTEX OF MONKEYS

KIYOSHI KURATA

Department of Neurophysiology, Tohoku University School of Medicine, Sendai 980, Japan

Recent experimental and clinical studies support the hypothesis that in both human and nonhuman primates the premotor cortex (PM) is either one or a set of motor fields in the cerebral cortex (see refs. *4, 20–22* for review). The premotor cortex is defined cytoarchitectonically as the lateral portion of Brodmann's area 6 of the agranular frontal cortex, thus located immediately rostral to the primary motor cortex (MI) and immediately lateral to the supplementary motor area (SMA). The contribution of the PM to motor control has long been ignored because electrical stimulations to the PM were ineffective to elicit muscle contraction, and because of its indistinct nature of motor deficits when excised. In contrast, the functional specialization of the MI and SMA in motor control has been the focus of many experimental studies, since the existence of both the MI and SMA has been well established by electrical stimulation studies. Recently, however, reports indicating that the PM is one of the motor fields have appeared following anatomical studies (*9, 11*), lesion studies (*12, 13*), regional cerebral blood flow studies (*14*), and single unit studies using awake, behaving monkeys (*2, 3, 5–8, 15, 19, 23*). This paper focuses on the results of the single unit studies.

I. FEATURES EMERGING FROM PM NEURONAL ACTIVITY IN BEHAVING PRIMATES

In neurophysiological studies using awake, behaving monkeys, behavioral tasks included a delay period during which an instruction stimulus for the forthcoming movement was presented while the animal withheld an overt movement. After this, a sensory trigger stimulus was provided to initiate the instructed movement. Among several patterns of PM neuronal discharges recorded while the monkeys were performing the motor tasks, two types of activity were found most frequent in the PM, thus providing a basis for the conclusion that the PM is one of the motor fields: 1) *set-related activity*, defined as sustained increases or decreases in the neuronal discharge rate after an instruction stimulus for a forthcoming movement is given until the movement is initiated; and 2) *movement-related activity*, defined as increases or decreases in the neuronal discharge rate immediately before movement onset, according to the nomenclature of Weinrich and Wise (*19*). Since the majority of the PM neurons with movement-related activity are limb-specific, and are topographically organized as well as in caudally adjacent MI (*6*), it has been argued that PM movement-related activity contributes to the initiation and execution of a specific limb movement. In contrast, set-related activity in the PM has been extensively studied by Wise and his colleagues (*10*, *19*, *23*) and by Godschalk (*2*, *3*), and it has been argued that this activity contributes to preparation for movement.

II. ROLES OF PM SET-RELATED ACTIVITY IN PREPARATION FOR MOVEMENT

On what basis does set-related activity reflect motor preparation, and then, in what aspect does PM set-related activity contribute to preparation for movement? Several examinations of PM set-related activity have been reported:

(1) Set-related activity has directional selectivity. Set-related neurons were active before the forelimb movement to one direction was initiated after the movement was instructed, and were inactive

before the movement to the opposite direction was initiated (*19*).

(2) A change in the instruction stimulus for the direction of forthcoming movements during the delay period also changed the set-related activity when this activity was directionally selective (*23*).

(3) The majority of PM neurons with set-related activity did not show a significant difference in their discharge rate when the instruction stimulus indicated the location of the target directly, or when it indicated the same target arbitrarily (*3*, *7*).

(4) The majority of PM neurons with set-related activity were equally active during the delay period when the location of the target was instructed by an externally-referenced sensory cue or by an internally-referenced cue (*8*, *15*).

Judging from the above, it seems that set-related activity of the PM is not dependent on the type of instruction cues and is closely linked to the forthcoming intended actions. Accordingly, it is hypothesized that set-related activity contributes to motor preparation in at least three aspects:

(1) *Motor programming.* Following the presentation of the instruction stimulus during the delay period, set-related activity emerged. Thus, it is tempting to propose that set-related activity contributes to motor programming by specifying which limb movement should be executed and how the movement should be carried out by determining various movement parameters necessary for execution of the intended action. It is well known that, in psychophysical experiments in humans, reaction time becomes significantly shorter in a two-choice motor task when the necessary action is previously instructed, compared to when it is not instructed. Set-related activity may play a role in shortening the reaction time if it contributes to motor programming. Further, it should be noted that the concept of motor programming may include various aspects of motor preparation not only for an immediate action, but also for sequential actions.

(2) *Inhibition of movement.* In one of the conditions in the neurophysiological studies, the monkeys were required to withhold a movement during the delay period until a trigger stimulus was presented to initiate the movement. During the delay period, set-related activity might be effective in suppressing the movement by sending an inhibitory output to lower motor centers.

(3) *Modulation of reflex action.* Modifiable reflex components with longer latency than spinal segmental reflex components have been attributed to the transcortical loop. Supporting this, the responsiveness of pyramidal tract neurons (PTNs) in the MI to proprioceptive input was found to be modified by behavioral set status (*1*). Set-related activity may be a driving force to modify the long loop reflex by sending excitatory or inhibitory output to PTNs in the MI.

Among these hypotheses, the first, regarding motor programming, is of particular interest when considering how a movement is programmed and prepared in the central nervous system. Thus, the motor programming hypothesis was examined in greater detail.

III. MOVEMENT PARAMETER PROGRAMMING REFLECTED IN PM SET-RELATED ACTIVITY

The findings on set-related activity led to a more specific question: is any movement parameter, such as direction, amplitude, velocity, or force, represented in set-related activity of the PM? So far, only one parameter, direction, has been reported to show a clear relationship to set-related activity; some PM neurons with set-related activity showed directional selectivity (*23*). Thus, it is not yet known if movement parameters other than direction are represented in the set-related activity of the PM, or if the PM set-related activity specifies multiple rather than single movement parameters so that an overall movement can be prepared. Prompted by these questions fundamental to understanding the nature of the PM set-set-related activity, PM neuronal activity was examined using macaque monkeys which were required to incorporate two motor instructions, one for direction and the other for amplitude, to be prepared for proper execution of forthcoming hand movements.

Neuronal activity was recorded from the PM of two Japanese monkeys (*Macaca fuscata*) performing a dually instructed motor task with four types of right-hand movement about the wrist joint: large flexion, small flexion, large extension, and small extension. The amplitudes of the large and small movements were 15° and 3° from the central hold zone, respectively. In order to instruct the four possible forthcoming movements during a delay period in which the monkeys withheld an overt movement, illumination of either the left or right red light emitting diode was used as an instruction stimulus (IS) for flexion and extension, respectively (direction IS). The 300 Hz and 1000 Hz tone signals were used as another IS for large and small movement, respectively (amplitude IS). After initiation of each trial by aligning the hand position on the central hold zone, the monkeys were required to withhold a movement for 3.0 sec to 3.8 sec (a delay period) by maintaining alignment of their hand position on the central hold zone until a visual trigger stimulus was presented. During the delay period, a direction IS and an amplitude IS were randomly selected and presented during different stages of the delay period in the above-mentioned order or in reversed order, so that the delay period was divided into two phases. The order of IS presentation was also randomized. Thus, either the direction or amplitude was instructed in the first half of the delay period, while the remaining parameter was instructed in the second half of the delay period. The first IS was presented 0.6 sec after trial initiation, then the second IS was presented 1.2 sec after the first IS presentation. The visual trigger stimulus was presented 1.2 sec to 2.0 sec after the second IS.

Since it was essential that the monkeys prepare for the forthcoming movements during the delay period so as to execute continuous programmed movements once the movements were initiated, the following five requirements had to be carried out in order to receive a reward as a reinforcement in each trial. First, the movement had to be initiated within 800 msec after a trigger stimulus is presented. Second, the initial movement direction had to be identical to that instructed. Third, the target zone should be reached within 500 msec after the movement was initiated. Fourth, the movement should not overshoot the target zone when small movements were required. Fifth, the position should be maintained for at least 300 msec within the target zone after the target acquisition by displacing the hand position.

After completion of training, the monkeys performed the task correctly on more than 90% of the trials, and all of the large and small movements were found to be continuous, without any disruption of the trajectory of movements. In the successful trials of the small movements, no overshooting movements from the targets were observed. Further, EMG activity of the forearm extensor and flexor, prime movers in the present task, did not change significantly or consistently during the delay periods. The extensor and the flexor muscles were active depending on the direction and the amplitude of the movements when they were initiated.

When the monkeys performed the task correctly, 54 PM set-related neurons were isolated and recorded long enough to compare the activity during the first and second delay periods in 8 conditions. Based on their discharge patterns in each phase of the delay periods, the neurons with set-related activity were classified into three types: 1) activity related to the direction only, termed *direction set-related activity*; 2) activity related to the amplitude only, termed *amplitude set-related activity*; 3) activity related to both the direction and the amplitude, termed *direction-plus-amplitude set-related activity*. The number of each type of set-related activity was 6, 2, and 46, respectively. Further, it is important to note that the neurons with the direction-plus-amplitude-set-related activity were most active after both the direction IS and amplitude IS were presented in the second half of the delay period.

The results indicate that the set-related activity of some PM neurons provide the code for the movement parameters most likely to be interpreted as both amplitude and direction. More importantly, since a majority of set-related neurons was most active after both the direction IS and the amplitude IS were presented, set-related activity of the PM, as a whole, may contribute to preparation for movement by integrating movement parameters necessary for execution of an intended action, rather than by specifying individual movement parameters. Thus, it is proposed that the PM set-related activity recorded in the present experiment represents the final stage of motor preparation containing all of the movement parameters.

IV. INTEGRATION OF CUES AND MOTOR PROGRAMMING

Since the majority of set-related neurons represent multiple movement parameters, the set-related activity seems to reflect the final form of motor programming. However, motor programming is not formed in the PM directly from externally- or internally-referenced cues. Rather, it is natural to suppose that there are many stages to the formation of a motor program in the central nervous system. Thus, it is important to speculate on these stages, and attempt to differentiate the motor preparation process into two stages:

(1) *Information extracting process.* Perceived sensory cues, in the case of externally-referenced behavior, are first analyzed in the primary sensory areas in the cerebral cortex. This information will be further processed in the sensory association cortex. The sensory cues used as an instruction stimulus may not have any direct link to the direction of the hand movement in these areas. Such cues should be processed into a more abstract form and the information, including movement parameters, necessary for the preparation and execution of movements must be extracted. This most likely occurs in the parietal association cortex, the temporal association cortex, the prefrontal cortex, or the motor loops involving the cerebellum and basal ganglia. Then, the cues might become the instructions available for motor programming. It may be also possible that the extracted information can be integrated in this process.

(2) *Motor programming process.* Extracted information should then be converted into the elements of the motor programs. Some possibilities are present in the form of conversion from extracted information to the motor program. First, if each piece of information for various movement parameters is separately extracted, then it is possible that the information can be converted into individual movement parameters. Second, the information integrated in the previous stage is directly converted into a motor program representing the multiple parameters. Third, several motor programs, each of which specifies a single movement parameter, are integrated to form a complete motor program.

V. COMPARISON OF SET-RELATED ACTIVITY IN THE OTHER AREAS

In the motor fields of the cerebral cortex, set-related activity was recorded not only in the PM but also in the MI and SMA (*16–18*). To date, it has been reported that set-related activity in the MI and SMA is directionally specific, thus representing direction as a movement parameter (*16*, *18*). However, it has not yet been investigated whether set-related activity in the MI and SMA represent movement parameters other than direction, or whether it represents multiple rather than single movement parameters, as proposed in this review for PM set-related activity. In the SMA, however, another aspect of set-related activity has been reported, since this activity in some cases did not exhibit a direct tight relationship with the movement parameters. It was suggested that SMA contributes to the sensory information selection process rather than to motor programming (*17*). If the sensory information selection process is equivalent to the information extracting process, as mentioned in the previous section, set-related activity in SMA could be regarded as the early stage of set-related activity in PM. Since the MI, PM, and SMA are interconnected, it is possible that the motor program which is represented in set-related activity is first generated in the SMA, then sent to the PM where the individual programs are integrated to form the complete program, and finally utilized in the MI.

SUMMARY

Recent neurophysiological studies indicate that the PM of primates plays an important role in motor programming as one aspect of motor preparation. Supporting this, it was found that the set-related activity of the PM, which has been reported to contribute to motor preparation, reflects multiple movement parameters necessary for execution of an intended action. Thus, the PM should be regarded as a distinct motor field where individual motor programs are integrated to form complete motor programs.

REFERENCES

1 Evarts, E.V. and Tanji, J. (1976). *J. Neurophysiol.* **39**, 1069–1080.
2 Godschalk, M., Lemon, R.N., Nijs, H.G.T., and Kuypers, H.G.J.M. (1985). *Behav. Brain Res.* **44**, 143–157.
3 Godschalk, M. and Lemon, R.N. (1985). *Soc. Neurosci.* Abstr. **11**, 74.
4 Humphrey, D.R. (1979). In *Posture and Movement*, ed. Talbot, R.E. and Humphrey, D.R., pp. 51–112. New York: Raven Press.
5 Kubota, K. and Hamada, I. (1978). *J. Physiol.* (*Paris*) **74**, 297–312.
6 Kurata, K., Okano, K., and Tanji, J. (1985). *Exp. Brain Res.* **60**, 188–191.

7 Kurata, K. and Wise, S.P. (1988a). *Exp. Brain Res.* **69**, 327-343.
8 Kurata, K. and Wise, S.P. (1988b). *Exp. Brain Res.* **72**, 237-248.
9 Martino, A.M. and Strick, P.L. (1987). *Brain Res.* **404**, 307-312.
10 Mauritz, K.-H. and Wise, S.P. (1986). *Exp. Brain Res.* **61**, 229-244.
11 Muakkassa, K.F. and Strick, P.L. (1978). *Brain Res.* **18**, 176-182.
12 Passingham, R.E. (1985). *Behav. Brain Res.* **18**, 175-185.
13 Passingham, R.E. (1988). *Exp. Brain Res.* **70**, 590-596.
14 Roland, P.E., Larsen, B., Lassen, N.A., and Skinhoj, E. (1980). *J. Neurophysiol.* **43**, 118-136.
15 Romo, R. and Schultz, W. (1987). *Exp. Brain Res.* **67**, 656-662.
16 Tanji, J. and Evarts, E.V. (1976). *J. Neurophysiol.* **39**, 1062-1068.
17 Tanji, J. and Kurata, K. (1985). *J. Neurophysiol.* **53**, 129-141.
18 Tanji, J., Taniguchi, K., and Saga, T. (1980). *J. Neurophysiol.* **43**, 60-68.
19 Weinrich, M. and Wise, S.P. (1982). *J. Neurosci.* **2**, 1329-1345.
20 Wiesendanger, M. (1981). In *Handbook of Physiology*, vol. II, ed. Brookhart, J.M., Mountcastle, V.B., Brooks, V.B, and Geiger, S.R., pp. 1121-1147. Bethesda, MD: American Physiological Society.
21 Wise, S.P. (1985). *Annu. Rev. Neurosci.* **8**, 1-19.
22 Wise, S.P. (1985). *Behav. Brain Res.* **18**, 79-88.
23 Wise, S.P. and Mauritz, K.-H. (1985). *Proc. R. Soc. Lond. B*, **223**, 331-354.

5

CORTICOSPINAL PROJECTIONS FROM THE MOTOR AREAS IN THE FRONTAL LOBE

RICHARD P. DUM AND PETER L. STRICK

Research Service, V. A. Medical Center, Departments of Neurosurgery and Physiology, SUNY Health Science Center at Syracuse, Syracuse, New York 13210, U.S.A.

Classically, the primary motor cortex has been viewed as the 'upper motoneuron' or 'final common pathway' for the central control of movement. However, the results of recent anatomical studies have indicated that the corticospinal system originates not only from the primary motor cortex, but also from multiple premotor areas in the frontal lobe (*e.g.*, ref. *4, 13, 25, 26, 30, 46*). These and other observations suggest that the central generation and control of movement may involve the activity of descending pathways from multiple cortical areas.

In several recent studies, we have examined the origin of cortical projections to the cervical and lumbar segments of the spinal cord using retrograde transport of wheat germ agglutinin conjugated to horseradish peroxidase (WGA-HRP) (*7, 8, 13, 26*). In this short report we will illustrate the origin of corticospinal projections from the premotor areas. To do this we will present the results of experiments in macaques with tracer injections into: 1) lower segments of the cervical spinal cord (C5–C8, Figs. 1 and 4A); 2) upper segments of the cervical cord (C2–C4, Fig. 2); and 3) lower lumbo-sacral segments (L5–S2, Fig. 4B).

In the course of our studies, we have found that some areas of the frontal lobe project differentially to upper or lower segments of the cervical cord. We will illustrate the most striking examples of this observation and discuss the potential significance of this result.

I. PREMOTOR AREAS ON THE MEDIAL WALL OF THE HEMISPHERE

Retrograde transport of tracer from cervical and lumbar segments of

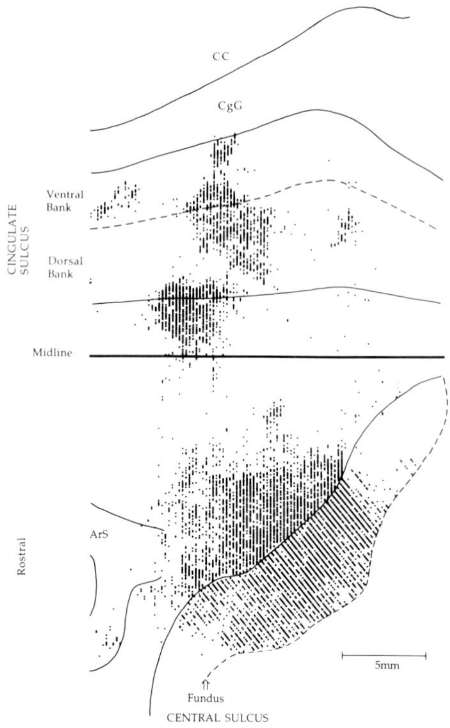

Fig. 1. The location of corticospinal neurons projecting to lower segments of cervical spinal cord (C5–C8). This diagram represents a flattened view of the frontal cortex which is reconstructed from individual coronal sections. Every fourth 50 μm section is charted and each labeled neuron is represented by a dot. The junction of the medial wall of the hemisphere with the lateral surface (*i.e.*, the midline) is used to align sections. The medial wall of the hemisphere is reflected upward and the cingulate sulcus is opened (see text and Fig. 3 for details). The anterior bank of the central sulcus is projected perpendicular to the mean angle of the sulcus with respect to the midline. The arcuate sulcus (ArS) and superior precentral sulcus (not indicated) are not opened. CgG, cingulate gyrus.

the spinal cord demonstrates that the premotor areas on the medial wall of the hemisphere have substantial corticospinal projections (Figs. 1, 2, 4, and 5). We display the medial wall of the hemisphere (Fig. 3) reflected upward in a manner similar to that of Woolsey (*56*, see also refs. *55, 57*). In addition, we have 'unfolded' the medial wall by separating it into 4 segments: 1) the medial aspect of the superior frontal gyrus; 2) the dorsal bank of the cingulate sulcus; 3) the ventral bank of the cingulate sulcus; and 4) the cingulate gyrus. The cytoarchitectonic borders between areas 4, 6 and subfields of areas 23 and 24 (Figs. 3 and 4) were determined using multiple criteria (*24, 48, 55*).

Three distinct groups of corticospinal neurons project from the premotor areas on the medial wall to the cervical spinal cord (Figs. 1, 2, and 4A). A large group of corticospinal neurons is located in

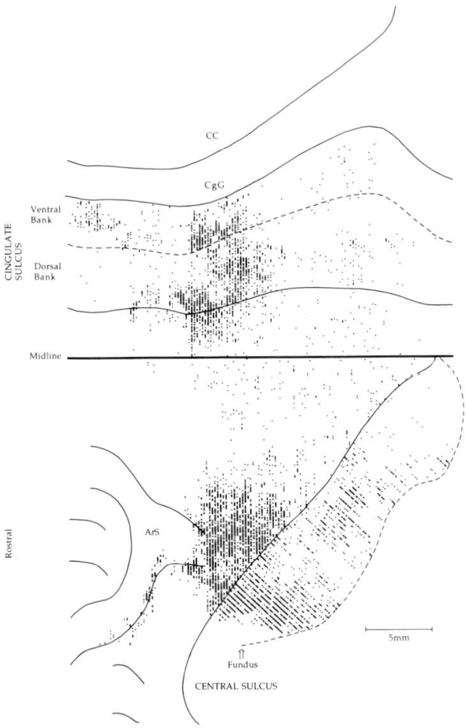

Fig. 2. The location of corticospinal neurons projecting to upper segments of cervical spinal cord (C2–C4). The method of reconstruction is the same as for Fig. 1.

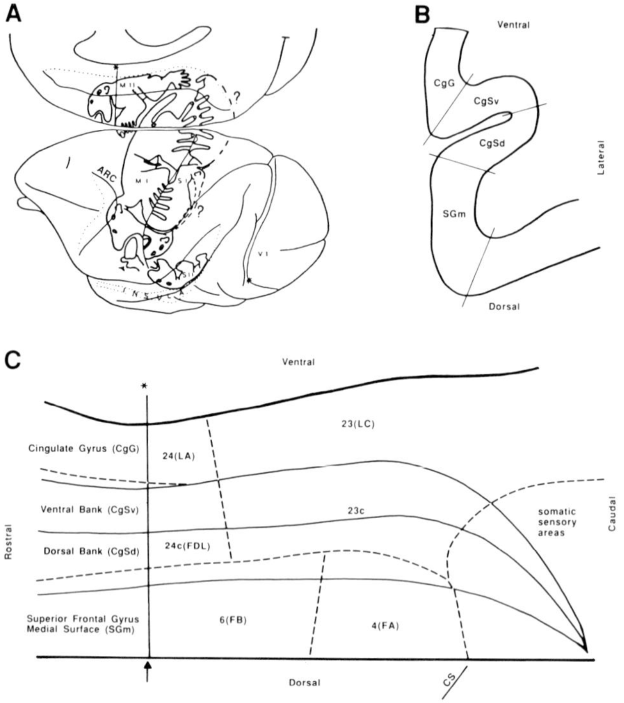

Fig. 3. Cortex on the medial wall of the hemisphere. A: maps of body representation in the cerebral cortex according to Woolsey (*56*). The medial wall of the hemisphere is reflected upwards to display the supplementary motor area (MII). We have adopted this convention for the other sections of this figure. Only the dorsal bank of the cingulate sulcus is opened in this diagram. B: a coronal section through the medial wall of the hemisphere at the level of the posterior extent of the arcuate sulcus (ARC). The level of this section is indicated by the vertical line in A marked by an asterisk. To unfold the medial wall, it was divided into 4 segments indicated by the thin solid lines through the section. The abbreviations in B are defined in C. C: unfolded map of the medial wall of the hemisphere. Sulcal borders are indicated by solid lines and cytoarchitectonic borders are indicated by dashed lines. The vertical line indicates the level of the coronal section shown in A and B. The arrow indicates the posterior extent of the arcuate sulcus. From Hutchins *et al.* (*13*).

area 6 on the medial aspect of the superior frontal gyrus at a level just caudal to the genu of the arcuate sulcus (arrow in Fig. 4A). A few of these corticospinal neurons are located on adjacent regions of the dorsal surface of the hemisphere and the dorsal bank of the cingulate sulcus. These corticospinal neurons lie within the region defined as the supplementary motor area (SMA) by Woolsey and his colleagues

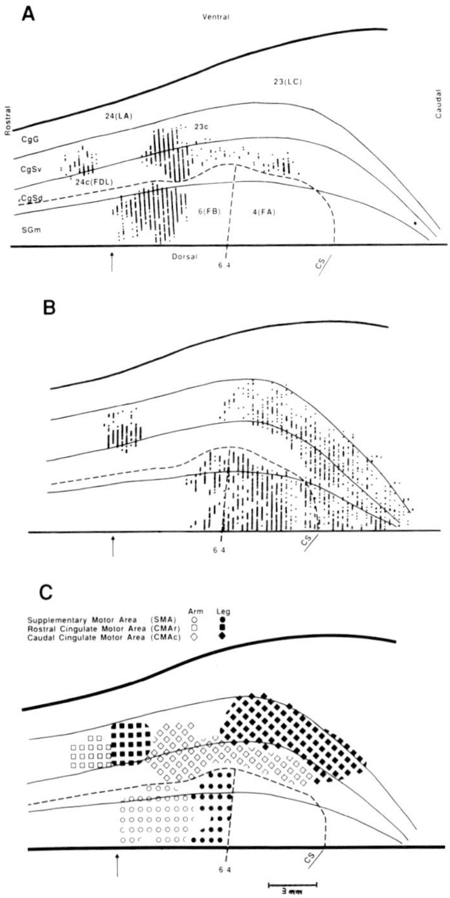

Fig. 4. Topographic origin of corticospinal projections from the medial wall. The unfolded maps of the medial wall are displayed using the conventions presented in Fig. 3. Arrows in A–C indicate the posterior extent of the arcuate sulcus. A: distribution of labeled neurons following tracer injections into C5–C8. B: distribution of labeled neurons following injections into L5–S2. C: labeling shown in A and B has been plotted on a single unfolded map using symbols: unfilled symbols, C5–C8 labeling; filled symbols, L5–S2 labeling; circles, labeling in the SMA; squares, labeling in the CMAr; diamonds, labeling in the CMAc. The labeled neurons in the hindlimb and tail representations in the primary motor cortex and various somatosensory areas are omitted from C to emphasize the pattern of projections from the premotor areas on the medial surface of the hemisphere. From Hutchins *et al.* (*13*).

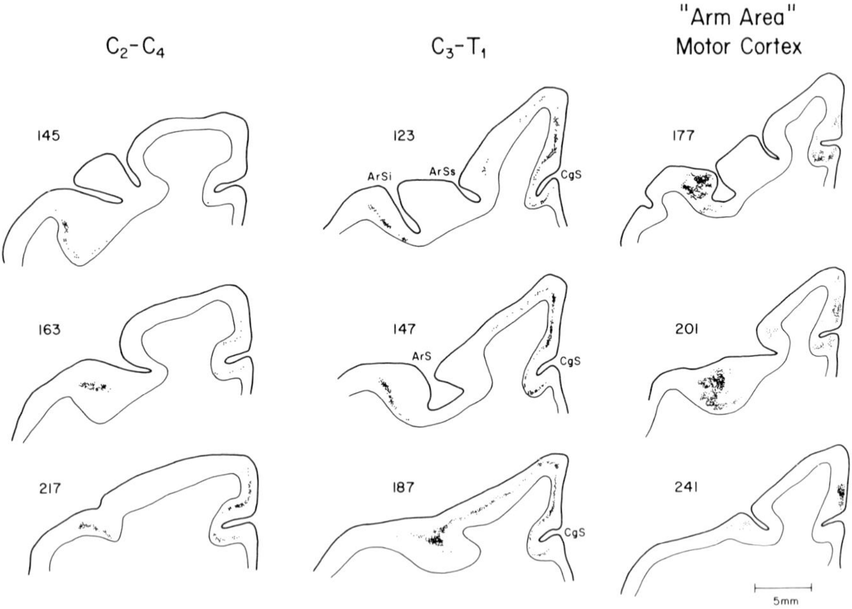

Fig. 5. Distribution of corticospinal neurons within the sulci of the frontal lobe. Labeled neurons are indicated by the small dots on these coronal sections. Note that injections of WGA-HRP into upper (C2–C4) or the upper and lower segments (C3–T1) of the cervical spinal cord result in substantial numbers of labeled neurons in the inferior limb of the arcuate sulcus (ArSi) and in the cingulate sulcus (CgS). The same regions of the ArSi and the medial wall contain labeled neurons following injections of WGA-HRP into the 'arm area' of the primary motor cortex. From Martino and Strick (*26*).

(*57*, see also refs. *24, 25, 28, 55, 56*). A second, small cluster of corticospinal neurons is located at rostral levels of the cingulate sulcus in a region termed FDL by Von Bonin and Bailey (*5*) and area 24c by Vogt (*48*). This cluster is found predominantly on the ventral bank of the sulcus at levels rostral to the genu of the arcuate sulcus. These corticospinal neurons lie within the region we have termed the rostral cingulate motor area (CMAr) (*13*). A third and more extensive group of corticospinal neurons is located at intermediate levels of the cingulate sulcus in a region termed LC by Von Bonin and Bailey (*5*) and area 23c by Vogt (*48*). In this area, neurons are found on both the dorsal and ventral banks of the sulcus beginning at levels caudal to the genu of the arcuate sulcus. These labeled neurons lie within the region we have termed the caudal cingulate motor area (CMAc) (*13*).

The medial wall of the hemisphere also contains 3 comparable groups of corticospinal neurons which project to the lumbo-sacral spinal cord (Fig. 4B). One group of corticospinal neurons is located in the SMA just anterior to the primary motor cortex. A second, small cluster of corticospinal neurons is located in the CMAr beginning at levels caudal to the genu of the arcuate sulcus (arrow in Fig. 4B). A third and more extensive group of corticospinal neurons is located in the CMAc largely on the ventral bank of the cingulate sulcus. These labeled neurons are found approximately at the anterior-posterior level of the 4/6 border. Large numbers of corticospinal neurons also originate from regions where the hindlimb and tail representations of the primary motor and somatic sensory cortex extend onto the medial wall of the hemisphere.

The topographic organization of corticospinal projections from the premotor areas on the medial wall is revealed by comparing the origin of cortical projections to lower cervical segments with the origin of projections to lower lumbar and sacral segments (Fig. 4C). We have overlapped the maps of labeled neurons from the animals illustrated in Fig. 4A, B. Clearly, in each premotor area, corticospinal projections to lower cervical segments are located rostral to those projecting to lower lumbar and sacral segments of spinal cord. This observation suggests that there are distinct arm and leg representations in the SMA, CMAc, and CMAr. It should be noted, however, that injections of tracers into different segments of the spinal cord can provide only a relatively gross measure of the topographic organization of corticospinal projections. Thus, the full extent of the somatotopic organization of the premotor areas on the medial wall of the hemisphere remains to be determined with alternative methods.

II. ARCUATE PREMOTOR AREA

Corticospinal projections originate from the arcuate premotor area (APA) which is located in a lateral part of area 6 (Figs. 1, 2, and 5) (*26*). Thus, all of the premotor areas which project directly to the 'arm' area of the primary motor cortex on the crest of the precentral gyrus (*i.e.*, APA, SMA, CMAc, and CMAr) (*29, 32, 41*) also project directly to cervical segments of the spinal cord (Fig. 5). The APA neurons which project to the spinal cord are located largely in the caudal bank of the arcuate sulcus. This finding is most clearly demonstrated by examining sections which pass through the sulcus (Fig. 5).

An important feature of the corticospinal system from the APA is that it does not project to all levels of the spinal cord. Tracer injections into lower cervical segments of spinal cord label only a small number of neurons in the APA (Fig. 1). Furthermore, no labeled neurons are found in this region after tracer injections into lumbo-sacral segments. Thus, the APA projection to the spinal cord terminates largely in upper cervical segments (Figs. 2 and 5).

III. PRIMARY MOTOR CORTEX

We have found that regions within the arm area of the primary motor cortex differ in the extent of their projection to cervical segments of the spinal cord (Figs. 1 and 2). Rostral and lateral portions of the arm area project to both upper and lower cervical segments. In contrast, a caudal portion of the arm area, which is buried in the anterior bank of the central sulcus, does not project to upper cervical segments, but is specifically targeted upon lower segments.

IV. DISCUSSION

A major result of these studies is that substantial numbers of corticospinal neurons originate from regions of the frontal lobe that lie outside of the primary motor cortex (see Figs. 1 and 2). For example, corticospinal neurons originate from the APA in lateral portions of area 6; from the SMA in more medial portions of area 6; and from the CMAr and CMAc in subfields of areas 24 and 23. In prior studies, we have shown that each of these regions projects directly to the 'arm' area of the primary motor cortex (*26*, *29*). Based on this connection, we have termed these cortical regions the 'premotor areas' of the frontal lobe (*26*, *29*, *36*, *41*, *42*, see also refs. *10*, *12*, *23*, *27*). Thus, our studies have shown that each of the premotor areas has dense projections not only to the primary motor cortex, but also to the spinal cord.

Our results indicate that the corticospinal projections from the premotor areas on the medial wall of the hemisphere are somatotopically organized. Projections to lower cervical segments of spinal cord originate from regions of the SMA, CMAr, and CMAc which are rostral to those which project to lower lumbo-sacral segments. The results of other studies using either anatomical or physiological techniques support this pattern of body representation (*6, 12, 24, 25, 27, 28*). They also provide evidence for separate face representations rostral to the arm representations in the SMA and CMAr (*6, 12, 29*). These observations suggest that each of these premotor areas contains at least a partial body map.

Recently, there has been a renewal of interest in exploring the motor functions of the premotor areas on the medial wall of the hemisphere (*e.g.*, refs. *35, 37, 51, 53, 54*). A complete discussion of the experiments, results and hypotheses concerning the participation of these cortical areas in the control of movement is clearly beyond the scope of this review. However, we would like to comment briefly on several functional considerations suggested by the present anatomical observations. Schell and Strick (*36*) recently proposed that the SMA is the major cortical site of termination for basal ganglia outputs related to limb movement (see also refs. *1, 52*). We believe that the SMA projections to the spinal cord may be particularly important because they provide the basal ganglia with a somatotopically organized route to the spinal cord.

Any discussion about the motor functions of the CMAr and CMAc is limited by the general lack of information regarding the anatomy and physiology of these regions. At present, the nomenclature that we have proposed for the CMAr and CMAc is meant *only* to reflect our working hypothesis that the 2 cingulate motor areas are directly involved in the control of movement in some as yet undetermined fashion (*e.g.*, refs. *9, 39, 50*). The proximity of the cingulate motor areas to the cingulate gyrus and the well known associations between cingulate cortex and the limbic system (see ref. *47* for a review) suggest that the corticospinal projections of the CMAr and CMAc represent a potential route by which the limbic system gains access to spinal cord mechanisms. We are currently performing anatomical experiments to investigate this possibility. However, it is important to note that the cingulate gyrus itself does not project directly to the spinal cord. Also, anatomical studies have not noted substantial connections between the cingulate gyrus and cortical regions buried within the cingulate sulcus (*47, 49*). Thus, the CMAr and CMAc may be separate from the limbic system and fundamentally different from the cortex on the cingulate gyrus.

Another important result of our studies is the demonstration that components of the corticospinal system have projections that are focused onto either upper or lower segments of the cervical spinal cord. The projection from the APA largely to upper cervical segments and the projection from the caudal part of the motor cortex to lower cervical segments are 2 striking examples of this observation. The existence of these distinct patterns of segmental projection suggests that these systems are concerned with controlling different aspects of movement. However, in the discussion to follow, we will argue that both systems have the potential to control distal limb movements.

Based on the level of termination, one might conclude that the projection from the APA to upper cervical segments influences spinal cord mechanisms concerned with the control of axial and proximal muscles. However, the motoneurons innervating axial and proximal muscles are located in lower, as well as, upper cervical segments (*33, 40*). Moreover, there is evidence that the interneurons which influence distal forelimb motoneurons are located throughout the cervical segments (*e.g.*, refs. *3, 14–16*). For example, in these studies on the cat spinal cord, Lundberg and his colleagues have identified a group of interneurons in upper cervical segments which form a disynaptic link between the corticospinal tract and forelimb motoneurons in lower cervical segments. Thus, even though the APA terminates primarily in upper cervical segments, it may project to spinal circuitry which influences the control of distal muscles.

This conclusion is supported by 3 additional observations. First, stimulation of the APA can evoke movements of the distal forelimb (*34*). Second, our findings indicate that the region of the APA which projects to upper cervical segments is reciprocally connected with a part of the primary motor cortex which contains the representation of the distal forelimb (see *26* for further references). Finally, the results of behavioral studies suggest that both the APA and those interneurons in upper cervical segments which are part of the disynaptic corticospinal pathway are involved in the guidance of forelimb movements in extrapersonal space (*e.g.*, refs. *2, 11, 34*).

In contrast to the APA, the caudal part of the primary motor cortex, by terminating in lower cervical segments, has a more direct access to distal forelimb motoneurons which are located solely in these segments (*e.g.*, refs. *17, 33, 40*). A large number of observations from prior studies support the concept that this region of primary motor cortex is involved in the control of distal forelimb musculature. For example, electrical stimulation of the caudal part of the primary motor cortex indicates that a motor representation of the hand is located in this region of motor cortex (*e.g.*, refs. *20, 38, 57*). Also, of all the cortical regions which project to the spinal cord, the caudal part of the primary motor cortex has the densest monosynaptic connections to distal limb motoneurons (see *19, 31* for References and Discussion). These and other observations, as well as the results of behavioral studies, have led Kuypers and his colleagues to suggest that the caudal part of the primary motor cortex is specifically concerned with the generation of relatively independent finger movements (see refs. *18, 19, 22*).

The focused nature of the corticospinal projection from the caudal part of the primary motor cortex distinguishes it from the remainder of the primary motor cortex. Prior physiological studies have reported other important differences between the rostral and caudal parts of the primary motor cortex. For example, the primary motor cortex of the squirrel monkey contains 2 spatially separate representations of the hand (*43, 44*). Neurons in the caudal representation received predominantly cutaneous input. In contrast, neurons in the rostral representation received predominantly deep input (muscles and/or joint). Comparable spatial segregation of deep and cutaneous input has been found in the forelimb and hindlimb representations of the primary motor cortex of macaques (*21, 45*). Based on the differences in somatosensory input to the 2 representations, Strick and Preston (*44*) proposed that the caudal representation is concerned with controlling hand movements which require tactile feedback for their execution and guidance. On the other hand, they proposed that the rostral representation is concerned with controlling hand movements which require kinesthetic feedback. Clearly, both anatomical and physiological studies indicate that the primary motor cortex is not a homogeneous field. Instead, we believe that the primary motor cortex should be viewed as containing at least 2 regions with distinct input-output characteristics and potentially different motor functions.

In summary, the corticospinal system of macaques consists of multiple pathways originating from primary motor and premotor areas of the frontal lobe. In fact, the contribution of the premotor areas to the corticospinal system is as substantial as that from the primary motor cortex. The premotor areas which project to the spinal cord also are interconnected with the primary motor cortex. Thus, each premotor area can influence the control of movement at both the cortical and spinal level. Our results indicate that even within the primary motor cortex, at least 2 components of the corticospinal system may be distinguished based on their patterns of segmental termination within cervical spinal cord. Based on these and other findings, we propose that multiple parallel pathways to the spinal cord from the primary motor cortex and the premotor areas in the frontal lobe participate in the central generation and control of movement.

SUMMARY

This report summarizes some of the results from our recent anatomical studies on the organization of the corticospinal system in the frontal lobe of monkeys. We used retrograde transport of wheatgerm agglutinin (WGA-HRP) to determine the origin of cortical projections to cervical and lumbar segments of the spinal cord. Our results indicate that the premotor areas in the frontal lobe have substantial projections to the spinal cord. These premotor areas are the same cortical regions which project directly to the primary motor cortex. They include the SMA on the superior frontal gyrus, 2 cingulate motor areas buried within the cingulate sulcus and the APA in the posterior bank of the arcuate sulcus. We also found that the corticospinal system from the primary motor cortex is divided into 2 components which are distinguished by their patterns of segmental termination within the cervical spinal cord. Thus, our studies have demonstrated that the frontal lobe contribution to the corticospinal system contains multiple components. Based on these and other findings, we propose that parallel pathways to the spinal cord from the primary motor cortex and the premotor areas in the frontal lobe participate in the central generation and control of movement.

Acknowledgments
This work has been supported in part through funds from the Veterans Administration Medical Research Service and Rehabilitation Research and Development Service and USPHS grants 02957 and 24328.

REFERENCES

1 Alexander, G.E., DeLong., M.R., and Strick, P.L. (1986). *Annu. Rev. Neurosci.* **9**, 357–381.
2 Alstermark, B., Lundberg, A., Norrsell, U., and Sybriska, E. (1981). *Exp. Brain Res.* **42**, 299–318.
3 Alstermark, B. and Sasaki, S. (1985). *Exp. Brain Res.* **59**, 353–364.
4 Biber, M.P., Kneisley, L.W., and LaVail, J.H. (1978). *Exp. Neurol.* **59**, 492–508.
5 Bonin, von G. and Bailey, P. (1947). *The Neocortex of Macaca mulatta*, vol. 5. Urbana, Ill: University of Illinois Press.
6 Brinkman, J. and Porter, R. (1979). *J. Neurophysiol.* **42**, 681–709.
7 Dum, R.P. and Strick, P.L. (1987). *Soc. Neurosci.* Abstr. **13**, 472.
8 Dum, R.P. and Strick, P.L. (1988). *Soc. Neurosci.* Abstr. **14**, 821.
9 Gemba, H., Sasaki, K., and Brooks, V.B. (1986). *Neurosci, Lett.* **70**, 223–227.
10 Ghosh, S., Brinkman, C., and Porter, R. (1987). *J. Comp. Neurol.* **259**, 424–444.
11 Godschalk, M., Lemon, R.N., Nijs, H.G.T., and Kuypers, H.G.J.M. (1981). *Exp. Brain Res.* **44**, 113–116.
12 Godschalk, M., Lemon, R.N., Kuypers, H.G.J.M., and Ronday, H.K. (1984). *Exp. Brain Res.* **56**, 410–424.
13 Hutchins, K.D., Martino, A.M., and Strick, P.L. (1988). *Exp. Brain Res.* **71**, 667–672.
14 Illert, M., Lundberg, A., and Tanaka, R. (1976). *Exp. Brain Res.* **26**, 521–540.
15 Illert, M., Lundberg, A., and Tanaka, R. (1977). *Exp. Brain Res.* **29**, 323–346.
16 Illert, M., Lundberg, A., Padel, Y., and Tanaka, R. (1978). *Exp. Brain. Res.* **33**,

101–130.
17 Jenny, A.B. and Inuki, J. (1983). *J. Neurosci.* **3**, 567–575.
18 Kuypers, H.G.J.M. and Brinkman, J. (1973). *Brain Res.* **24**, 29–48.
19 Kuypers, H.G.J.M. (1981). In *Handbook of Physiology*, vol. II, ed. Brooks, V.B., pp. 597–666. Bethesda, MD: American Physiological Society.
20 Kwan, H.C., MacKay, W.A., Murphy, J.T., and Wong, Y.C. (1978). *J. Neurophysiol.* **41**, 1120–1131.
21 Lamour, Y., Jennings, V.A., and Solis, H. (1980). *Soc. Neurosci.* Abstr. **6**, 158.
22 Lawrence, D.G. and Kuypers, H.G.J.M. (1968). *Brain* **91**, 1–14.
23 Leichnetz, G.R. (1986). *J. Comp. Neurol.* **254**, 460–492.
24 Macpherson, J., Marangoz, C., Miles, T.S., and Wiesendanger, M. (1982a). *Exp. Brain Res.* **45**, 410–416.
25 Macpherson, M., Wiesendanger, M., Marangoz, C., and Miles, T.S. (1982b). *Exp. Brain Res.* **48**, 8–88.
26 Martino, A.M. and Strick, P.L. (1987). *Brain Res.* **404**, 307–312.
27 Matsumura, M. and Kubota, K. (1979). *Neurosci. Lett.* **11**, 241–246.
28 Mitz, A.R. and Wise, S.P. (1987). *J. Neurosci.* **7**, 1010–1021.
29 Muakkassa, K.F. and Strick, P.L. (1979). *Brain Res.* **177**, 176–182.
30 Murray, E.A. and Coulter, J.D. (1981). *J. Comp. Neurol.* **195**, 339–365.
31 Phillips, C.G. and Porter, R. (1977). *Corticospinal Neurones: Their Role in Movement.* New York: Academic Press.
32 Primrose, D. and Strick, P.L. (1985). *Soc. Neurosci.* Abstr. **11**, 1274.
33 Reed, A.F. (1940). *J. Comp. Neurol.* **72**, 187–206.
34 Rizzolatti, G. and Gentilucci, M. (1988). In *Neurobiology of Neocortex*, ed. Rakic, P. and Singer, W., pp. 269–284. New York: John Wiley & Sons Ltd.
35 Roland, P.E., Larsen, B., Lassen, N.A., and Skinhoj, E. (1980). *J. Neurophysiol.* **43**, 118–136.
36 Schell, G.R. and Strick, P.L. (1984). *J. Neurosci.* **4**, 539–560.
37 Schlag, J. and Schlag-Rey, M. (1987). *J. Neurophysiol.* **57**, 179–200.
38 Sessle, B.J. and Wiesendanger, M. (1982). *J. Physiol.* **323**, 245–265.
39 Showers, M.J.C. (1959). *J. Comp. Neurol.* **112**, 231–287.
40 Sprague, J.M. (1948). *Am. J. Anat.* **82**, 1–26.
41 Strick, P.L. (1985). *Behav. Brain Res.* **18**, 107–123.
42 Strick, P.L. (1988). In *Advances in Neurology*, vol. 47, ed. Waxman, S.G., pp. 293–312. New York: Raven Press.
43 Strick, P.L. and Preston, J.B. (1982a). *J. Neurophysiol.* **48**, 139–149.
44 Strick, P.L. and Preston, J.B. (1982b). *J. Neurophysiol.* **48**, 150–159.
45 Tanji, J. and Wise, S.P. (1981). *J. Neurophysiol.* **45**, 467–481.
46 Toyoshima, K. and Sakai, H. (1982). *J. Hinforsch.* **23**, 257–269.
47 Vogt, B.A. (1985). In *Cerebral Cortex*, vol. 4, ed. Peters, A. and Jones, E.G., pp. 89–149. New York: Plenum.
48 Vogt, B.A., Pandya, D.N., and Rosene, D.L. (1987). *J. Comp. Neurol.* **262**, 256–270.

49 Vogt, B.A. and Pandya, D.N. (1987). *J. Comp. Neurol.* **262**, 271–289.
50 Ward, A.A. (1948). *J. Neurophysiol.* **11**, 13–24.
51 Wiesendanger, M. (1981). In *Handbook of Physiology. The Nervous System*, vol. 2, Part 2, ed. Brooks, V.B., pp. 1121–1148. Bethesda, MD: American Physiological Society.
52 Wiesendanger, R. and Wiesendanger, M. (1985). *Exp. Brain Res.* **59**, 91–104.
53 Wise, S.P. (1985). *Annu. Rev. Neurosci.* **8**, 1–19.
54 Wise, S.P. and Strick, P.L. (1984). *Trends Neurosci.* **7**, 442–446.
55 Wise, S.P. and Tanji, J. (1981). *J. Comp. Neurol.* **195**, 433–442.
56 Woolsey, C.N. (1958). In *Biological and Biochemical Bases of Behavior*, ed. Harlow, H.F. and Woolsey, C.N., pp. 63–81. Madison, WI: Univ. Wisconsin Press.
57 Woolsey, C.N., Settlage, P.H., Meyer, D.R., Sencer, W., Pinto Hamuy, T., and Travis, A.M. (1952). *Res. Publ. Assoc. Res. Nerv. Ment. Dis.* **30**, 238–264.

CONTRIBUTION OF THE CEREBELLUM, BASAL GANGLIA AND THALAMUS TO NEURAL PROGRAMMING

6

MOTOR PROGRAMME FOR VOLUNTARY MOVEMENT IN THE CEREBRO-CEREBELLAR NEURONAL CIRCUIT

KAZUO SASAKI* AND HISAE GEMBA

Department of Physiology, Institute for Brain Research, Faculty of Medicine, Kyoto University, Kyoto 606, Japan

I. CEREBRO-CEREBELLAR INTERACTION IN LEARNING AND COMPENSATING PROCESSES OF CONDITIONED HAND MOVEMENT

Intended movements are manifested by descending neuronal impulses impinging upon cranial and/or spinal motoneurones where segmental mechanisms are integrated together with the descending impulses. One of the major pathways for transmission of the impulses originates in the motor cortex to which the convergence comes not only from other cortical areas through association and commissura fibres but also from the basal ganglia and the cerebellum *via* thalamo-cortical afferents. Based on accumulated knowledge from previous morphological and physiological studies (*1*, *2*) as well as our own investigations (*13*, *14*), Sasaki drew a diagram of cerebro-cerebellar interconnections in monkeys (Fig. 1A, B) (*5*), and started chronic experiments on monkeys with Gemba and other associates. They recorded field potentials from various cortical areas in learning processes of visually- or auditory-initiated reaction-time hand move-

* Present address: Institute for Brain Research, Faculty of Medicine, Kyoto University, Kyoto 606, Japan.

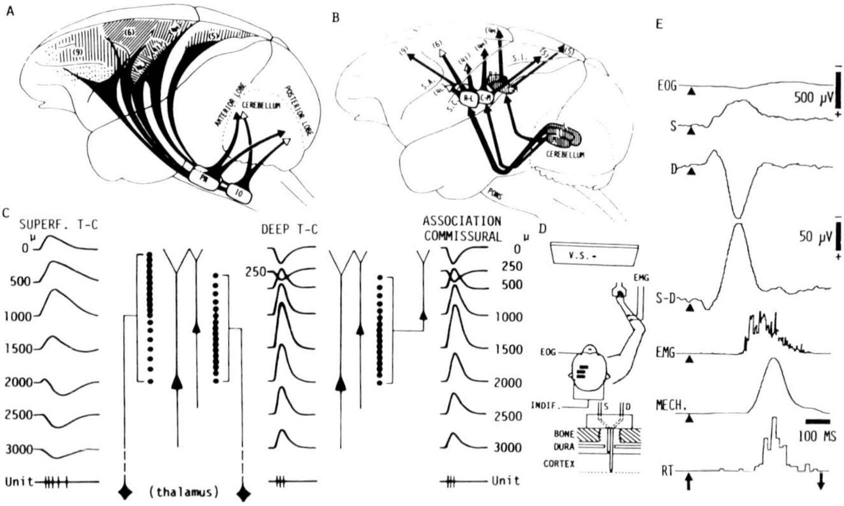

Fig. 1. A and B: diagrams of cerebro-cerebellar interconnections in monkeys. Numbers indicate the different cortical areas after Brodmann. Area 4 is divided into lateral (4L), intermediate (4I) and medial (4M) parts. PN, pontine nuclei; IO, inferior olive; S.A., arcuate sulcus; S.C., central sulcus; S.I., intraparietal sulcus; M, I, L, medial, interpositus, lateral nuclei of the cerebellum. R-L, C-M, two nuclear complexes of the thalamus. C: diagrams of laminar field potentials in the cortex by the two thalamo-cortical (superficial and deep T-C) and cortico-cortical (association and commissural) inputs. Numbers indicate the depth from the cortical surface in μm. Unit, schematic pattern of firing of cortical pyramidal neurone. The presumed excitatory synaptic terminals on apical dendrites of cortical pyramidal neurones in layers III and V are diagramatically shown by dots for the three afferent inputs. Laminar field potentials are attributed to electrical dipoles generated in pyramidal neurones by the EPSPs. D: diagrams of the methods of chronic experiments with monkeys (*Macaca fuscata*). Silver needle electrodes (about 200 μm in diameter), insulated except for their pointed tips, were placed on the surface (S) and at 2.0-3.0 mm depth (D) respectively in various cortical areas of both hemispheres and fixed to the bone by dental cement (see lower part of D). Each S and D electrode refers to an indifferent electrode placed in the bone behind the ear (INDIF). The monkey was presented with a light stimulus of the diode emitting two different colours (VS) and charged with lifting a lever by wrist extension within the duration of the light stimulus (usually about 500 msec). E: examples of EOG, cortical field potentials (S, D, S-D) in the forelimb motor cortex contralateral to the operant hand, mechanogram of lever movement (MECH) and reaction time histogram (RT) (16 msec bin) are presented. EMG was led bipolarly from the skin over wrist extensor muscles and rectified. They were aligned 100 times at the onset of visual stimulus (upward arrows and triangles); end of the stimulus is shown by a downward arrow. Calibration of 500 μV for EOG and 50 μV for cortical potentials. 100 msec time scale for all traces. (Modified from Sasaki (*5*)).

ments with chronically implanted electrodes in these areas (*4, 6*).

In those experiments, several main points were substantiated (see ref. *10*): 1. The process of 'recognition learning' for associating the external stimulus with the hand movement is accompanied by increasing activity in the association cortices and the premotor cortices of both hemispheres. For visually-initiated movement, the prefrontal, premotor and prestriate cortices are predominantly activated (*6*) (Fig. 2-I–III), whereas for auditory-initiated movement, the auditory association cortices appear to be more excited than the prefrontal and premotor cortices (*3, 4*). 2. The process of late learning stage in which the movement becomes faster and less variable in its timing, called 'skill learning', is promoted by recruiting the cerebro-cerebellar interaction (*4, 6, 7*). This is seen by gradual increase of the surface-negative, depth-positive (s-N, d-P) field potential in the forelimb area of motor cortex contralateral to the operant hand (Fig. 2III, IV, row E; see Fig. 1E). This potential has been proved to be due mainly to EPSP currents in the superficial part of apical dendrites of pyramidal neurones in the cortex and to be generated by the neuronal volley *via* the cerebello-thalamo-cortical pathway (*5, 6, 11*). The hemispherical part of the cerebellum (posterior lobe, neocerebellum) is essential for the acquisition of fast and appropriate timing of the movement, an element of skillfulness (*6*). 3. With cerebellar hemispherectomy in a well-trained monkey, the reaction-time movement is degraded to the state prior to skill learning; it can be performed although it is slow, irregular, and awkward. The compensatory motor function of the somatosensory cortex was found to replace, though incompletely, the motor cortex rendered dysfunctional by the cerebellectomy at least for several weeks after the operation (*8*) (substitution compensation). When the cerebellectomy includes both dentate and interpositus nuclei, prolonged reaction times recover little. However, when only the dentate nucleus is removed, prolonged and unstable reaction times are restored to the preoperative state and the s-N, d-P potential in the forelimb motor area reappears, presumably because of the compensatory participation of the preserved interpositus nucleus for the dentate function which would exert, if present (*11*). In this case, the recovery of reaction time and potential requires further training of several weeks

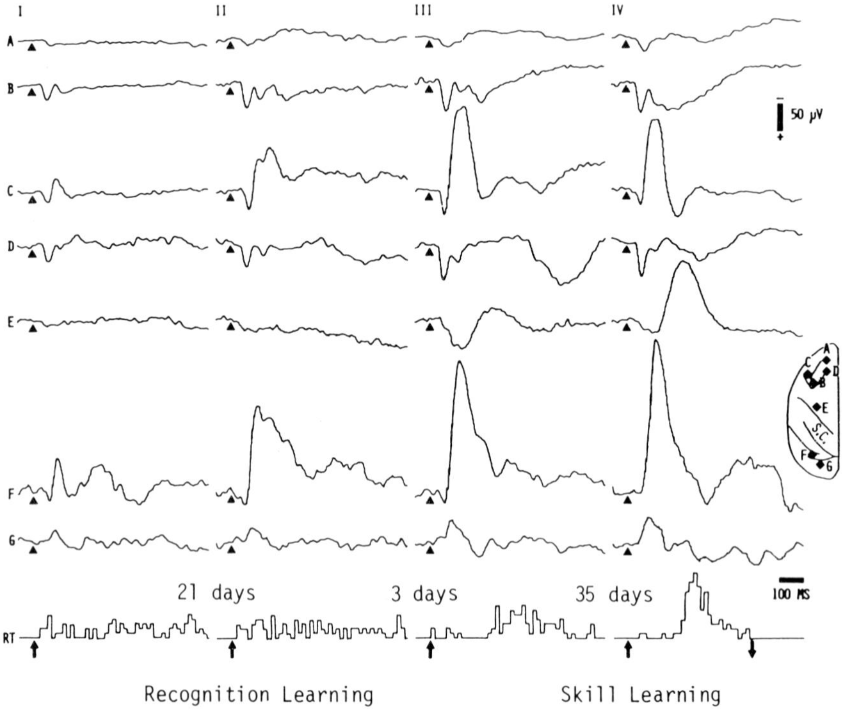

Fig. 2. Movement-related field potentials (S–D, surface minus depth) in seven cortical loci on the left hemisphere of a monkey learning the visually-initiated reaction-time movement of the right hand. Columns I–IV reflect four sessions at different stages. I was taken in the second session, II 21 days after I, III 3 days after II, and IV 35 days after III. Potentials were averaged 100 times from every session for respective cortical loci indicated by alphabetical symbols in the inset diagram and each row of records. The stimulus was given for 900 msec at stages I–III but 510 msec at IV. Only the movements which occurred during the light stimulus were counted in RTs and averaged potentials (the latter part of 900 msec is curtailed in columns I–III). Movements were aligned by the stimulus onset pulse as indicated by triangles and upward arrows, a downward arrow showing the end of the 510 msec stimulus. Calibration of 50 μV for all potentials and 100 msec for all traces. (Sasaki and Gemba (*6*)).

similar to the skill learning in the normal naive animal (relearning compensation) (see ref. *10*).

In this article, we will take up field potential in the motor cortex which is, as mentioned above, considered to represent the EPSP current in the cortex generated by the neuronal volley through the cerebellum and the thalamus. The potential appears to comprise a motor command exciting the motor cortex to initiate the movement. This is gradually built in the process of skill learning, as reaction times become shorter and less variable (Fig. 2III, IV). Furthermore, it was recently found that latent time of the potential can be shifted to a certain extent by suppressor action due to stimulation of the special prefrontal loci (*12*). It is interesting to note that the latency shift occurs without much change of its configuration or action, as will be shown below. This supports our assumption that the potential represents a kind of consolidated motor command transmitted through the cerebello-thalamo-cerebral neuronal circuit, and suggests that the command consists of a neuronal programme acquired in the processes of motor learning.

II. PREFRONTAL LOCI PRODUCING 'NO-GO POTENTIAL' AND SUPPRESSOR ACTION BY STIMULATING THE LOCI UPON THE MOTOR COMMAND: MOTOR PROGRAMME REVEALED

In studying activities of the prefrontal cortex related to the go/no-go discriminative hand movement task with different colour light stimuli, we found a field potential in the prefrontal cortex specific to the no-go reaction, called 'no-go potential' (*9*). This potential is composed of s-N, d-P deflections in the caudal part of the dorsal bank in the principal sulcus and also in the ventrolateral corner of the inferior convexity of the prefrontal cortex (A and B in Fig. 3-II). It appears at a latency of 85–150 msec after the onset of no-go visual stimulus and lasts for 50–150 msec or so. The specificity of the potential to the no-go reaction was confirmed by the reversal experiment of go and no-go stimuli (*9*). The potential appears, disappears, and reappears in accordance with acquisition, confusion, and relearning of the discrimination task in the reversal experiment. Therefore, the potential is presumed to be related to the judgement not to move the hand and/or the suppressor action upon motor execution. Confirmation of the presumed suppressor action was gained in the experiment of stimulating the prefrontal loci (*12*).

A train of brief electrical pulses was delivered to the prefrontal loci producible of the no-go potential in both hemispheres, being applied bipolarly through the electrodes implanted on the surface

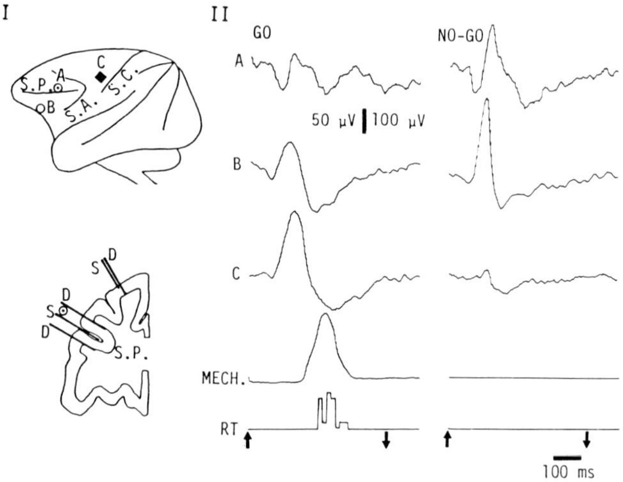

Fig. 3. 'No-go potential' in the prefrontal cortex. I: diagrams showing arrangement of recording electrodes in the principal sulcus (SP) and the dorsolateral and lateral part of the prefrontal area (lateral view and frontal section of the left hemisphere). Three electrodes about 2.5 mm apart were inserted in the sulcus parallel with each other; one of these (S) was used to record from the surface of dorsal and ventral banks in the sulcus, and the others (D) to record from the depths of respective banks. II: S–D potentials in the dorsal bank of the principal sulcus (A) (circle with a dot in centre in I), in the ventrolateral corner of the inferior convexity (B) (open circle in I) and in the forelimb motor cortex (C) (filled square in I) were aligned 20 times respectively at the onsets of go (green light) and no-go (red light) visual stimuli (GO and NO-GO columns). MECH and RT are shown for the 20 go and 20 no-go trials. The go and no-go signals were presented at irregular intervals of 5–10 sec and in random order. Note upward deflections of potentials (surface-negative, depth-positive no-go potentials) in the loci A and B on no-go trials when no movements occurred as revealed in MECH and RT. 50 μV calibration for B and C rows; A row was amplified twice as much as B and C rows. 100 msec scale for all traces.

(anode) and at 2.0–3.0 mm depth (cathode) of respective loci which were originally used to record the potential (S and D electrodes in Fig. 3-I and Fig. 1D). The electrical stimulus was given at various times after the onset of go visual stimulation (Fig. 4). The uppermost row of Fig. 4 shows the control records on the go visual stimulus without any electrical stimulation, *i.e.*, a field potential (S—D, surface minus depth potential) in the forelimb area of the motor cortex (FM) contralateral to the moving hand, a mechanogram (MECH) through a transducer attached to a lever and a reaction time histogram (RT)

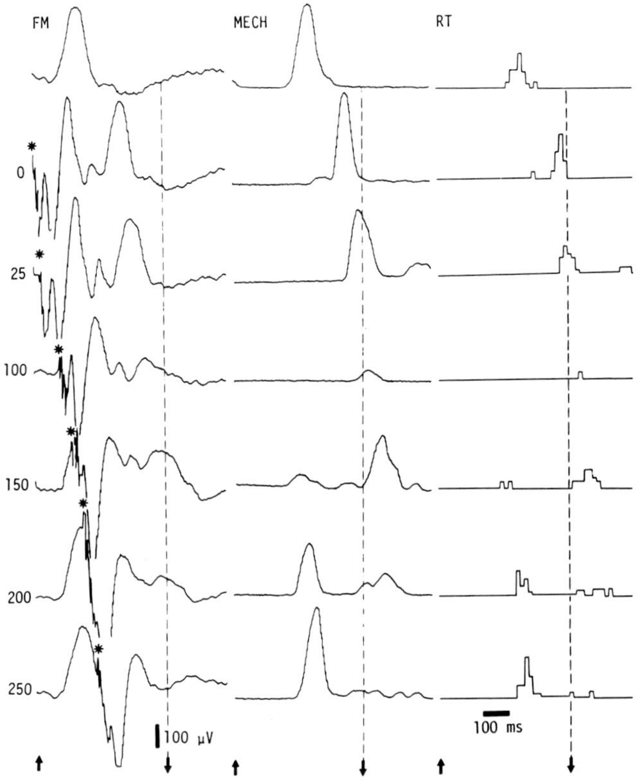

Fig. 4. Effects of electrical stimulation of the loci A and B of both hemispheres (Fig. 3) upon the premovement potential (S–D) in the forelimb motor cortex (FM), MECH, and RT. A train of electrical pulses (asterisks) was given at various times (0–250 msec) after the onset of go visual stimulus (beginning of every trace marked by upward arrows). The end of visual stimulus is shown by downward arrows and broken line. Each row was the average of 20 samples in one session by the onset pulse of visual stimulus. For further explanation, see text. 100 μV calibration for FM column and 100 msec scale for all traces.

with 16 msec bins. FM and MECH were aligned 20 times at the onset time of go visual stimulus, as indicated respectively by upward and downward arrows, broken lines denoting the end of the stimulus (visual stimulus of about 500 msec duration).

The upward deflexion in the control FM record (uppermost row, FM) represents the s-N, d-P field potential generated mainly by EPSP currents in pyramidal neurones of the forelimb motor cortex through the cerebello-thalamo-cortical pathway as mentioned above. It precedes the reaction-time hand movement (MECH and RT) by a certain latent time (see also Fig. 1E; C, GO in Fig. 3-II) and activates the motor area to induce the movement. Under such circumstances, the electrical stimulation of the prefrontal loci was given and resulted in delay and cancelling of the movement, as exemplified in Fig. 4 (second to bottom rows). A train of pulses (1 msec duration, 3 msec interval, 10 pulses, 0.7 mA) (the beginning is marked by asterisk) was given at various times after the onset of go visual stimulus as shown for 0, 25, 100, 150, 200, and 250 msec. The stimulus at 0 msec (second row designated by 0 to the left) induced a complicated stimulus artefact that was immediately followed by downward and upward deflections. At about 270 msec after the stimulus, an upward potential appeared and looked similar to the cerebellar-mediated potential in the control record (uppermost row). The stimulus at 25 msec (third row, 25) further shifted the upward potential by about 25 msec. MECHs and RTs revealed that the stimuli at 0 and 25 msec after the onset of visual stimulus delayed the movement by about 160 and 160+25 msec. These data can be most reasonably interpreted as follows: a neuronal volley mediated by the cerebellum and the thalamus to the motor cortex is delayed by the electrical stimulation for about 160 msec and 160+25 msec without appreciable deformation and dysfunction, so that the movement is simply postponed accordingly by approximately the same time.

The electrical stimulus given at 100 msec after the go visual stimulus induced a different effect upon the movement, *i.e.*, it cancelled the movement except for that portion which occurred after the end of visual stimulus (failure to obtain a reward) (see MECH and RT in Fig. 4, fourth row). Such a cancelling action was observed by the stimulation given at 75–125 msec after the onset of go visual stimulus. Interestingly, this time range corresponds to the latency of no-go potential (85–110 msec in this monkey) with a time lag (see Fig. 3-II A and B, NO-GO). The electrical stimulus delivered at 150 and 200 msec after the visual stimulus curtailed the cerebellar-mediated potential in accord with the timing of the electrical stimuli; it allowed certain movements that occurred at relatively earlier latencies among the 20 samples averaged in these records to be manifested at the reaction times in a normal range, but postponed the rest of the movements. The stimulus at 250 msec revealed that the suppressor effect was almost over and only a few movements were delayed.

These results imply that the electrical stimulus to the prefrontal loci producing the no-go potential induces two kinds of actions on the movement, *i.e.*, delaying and cancelling. Site and mechanism of the actions are not yet known. As it concerns the nature of no-go potential itself, the cancelling action seems an interesting subject to study. On the other hand, the delaying action appears instructive for interpreting the neuronal volley transmitted through the cerebellum and the thalamus to the motor cortex. The phenomenon of latency shift by the delaying action suggests that the neuronal volley manifested as the s-N, d-P potential (EPSP currents) in the forelimb motor cortex contains a motor command, *i.e.*, a neuronal programme fairly well organized through the cerebellum and the thalamus. How such a programme can be organized through the cerebro-cerebellar interaction remains an important subject to be investigated.

SUMMARY

1. The main points of our previous studies on changes of cortical field potentials in monkeys during processes of motor learning of visually- and auditory-initiated reaction-time hand movement and during those of compensation after cerebellar hemispherectomy were very briefly reviewed.

2. The aspect of the particular field potential in the forelimb motor cortex, which is composed of EPSP currents in the cortical pyramidal neurones generated by the neuronal volley transmitted through the cerebello-thalamo-cortical pathway was taken up. It was suggested to include the motor programme conveyed *via* the pathway, referring to experimental data of the delaying action of prefrontal stimulation upon the potential and movement.

REFERENCES

1 Allen, G.I. and Tsukahara, N. (1974). *Physiol. Rev.* **54**, 957–1004.

2 Evarts, E.V. and Thach, W.T. (1969). *Annu. Rev, Physiol.* **31**, 451–498.

3 Gemba, H. and Sasaki, K. (1987). *Exp. Brain Res.* **65**, 649–657.
4 Gemba, H. and Sasaki, K. (1988). *Exp. Brain Res.* **70**, 43–49.
5 Sasaki, K. (1979). In *Cerebro-Cerebellar Interactions*, ed. Massion, J. and Sasaki, K., pp. 105–124. Amsterdam: Elsevier/North-Holland Biomedical Press.
6 Sasaki, K. and Gemba, H. (1982). *Exp. Brain Res.* **48**, 429–437.
7 Sasaki, K. and Gemba, H. (1983). *Brain Res.* **277**, 41–46.
8 Sasaki, K. and Gemba, H. (1984). *Exp. Brain Res.* **56**, 532–538.
9 Sasaki, K. and Gemba, H. (1986). *Exp. Brain Res.* **64**, 603–606.
10 Sasaki, K. and Gemba, H. (1987). *Acta Neurochirurgica* (Suppl.) **41**, 18–28.
11 Sasaki, K., Gemba, H., and Mizuno, N. (1982). *Exp. Brain Res.* **46**, 29–36.
12 Sasaki, K., Gemba, H., and Tsujimoto, T. (1989). *Brain Res.*, in press.
13 Sasaki, K., Kawaguchi, S., Oka, H., Sakai, M., and Mizuno, N. (1976). *Exp. Brain Res.* **24**, 495–507.
14 Sasaki, K., Oka, H., Kawaguchi, S., Jinnai, K., and Yasuda, T. (1977). *Exp. Brain Res.* **29**, 419–428.

7

THE NEOSTRIATAL MOSAIC: COMPARTMENTAL ORGANIZATION OF CORTICOSTRIATAL INPUT, STRIATONIGRAL OUTPUT AND DOPAMINERGIC FEEDBACK SYSTEMS

CHARLES R. GERFEN

Laboratory of Cell Biology, National Institute of Mental Health, Bethesda, Maryland 20892, U.S.A.

The basal ganglia provide a major neural system through which the cortex affects behavior. While it is clear that there is a major role for this sytem in motor function, it is becoming equally clear that virtually all aspects of behavior are affected by the basal ganglia. For example, Hikosaka and Wurtz (*20*) have demonstrated that the output systems of the basal ganglia not only encode movement related information, but that this information is also coupled to memory and motivationally contingent cues. In this sense the basal ganglia may be considered a cognitive motor system, in which movement, memory and emotional functions are integrated. That all areas of the cortex provide inputs to the basal ganglia argues for such an integrative function. By providing information on the organization of inputs, intrinsic connections and outputs, neuroanatomical studies aid in defining the possible nature of this integration.

In broad outline the major connections of the basal ganglia may be summarized as follows. The cortex provides a major, excitatory input to the striatum (*23*), which is composed of the caudate, putamen, and nucleus accumbens. The striatum, in turn, provides inhibitory input to tonically active neurons in the globus pallidus and substantia nigra (*4*) which are the major output nuclei of the basal ganglia. These nuclei provide inputs to the thalamus and midbrain motor areas, including the superior colliculus (*5*) and pedunculopontine nucleus. Feedback to the striatum is provided by the substantia nigra and the thalamus. Thus the striatum may be viewed as the central component of this sytem. Some 95% of the neurons in the striatum are of one morphologic type, the medium spiny projection neuron (*22*). These neurons provide the major output of the striatum while most of the rest of the neuronal cell types are intrinsic neurons with axonal connections that remain confined to the striatum.

A major concept to emerge over the past decade is that the striatum is a mosaic of two compartments, termed the patches and matrix. While the compartmental organization of the striatum was initially related to neurochemical heterogeneity (*16*, *18*, *25*), it is now evident that the patch and matrix compartments are formed by the segregation of two populations of medium spiny neurons that have distinct connections (*9*, *10*, *12*). The organization of these connections suggests that the patch and matrix compartments provide parallel, segregated but interactive input-output pathways. My studies now suggest that the compartmental organization of the striatum is related to the laminar organization of the cortex. A description of the studies that lead to this conclusion provides new concepts of the nature of the integrative capacity of the basal ganglia.

I. STRIATONIGRAL OUTPUT SYSTEMS

As many as 95% of striatal neurons are of one cell type, the medium spiny neuron (*22*). These neurons have a cell soma approximately 20 μM in diameter from which radiates relatively unbranched dendrites that are densely studded with spines. The dendritic arbors cover an area approximately 200–250 μm in diameter. This neuron provides the major output of the striatum, and is the major target of most of the extrinsic afferents of the striatum (*17*, *28*). Thus the function of the striatum is intimately related to the organization of the connections of these neurons (see ref. *11* for review). Cortical inputs to these neurons are excitatory, probably using glutamate as a transmitter, and synapse on the heads of the dendritic spines. Dopaminergic inputs to these neurons are directed to the necks of the spines or to the interspine segments. Additionally, these neurons receive inputs from neighboring medium spiny neurons, through local axon collaterals, whose spread roughly matches the dendritic arborization of the issuing neuron. Intrinsic neurons containing either acetylcholine, somatostatin or parvalbumin also provide inputs to these neurons.

Medium spiny neurons are segregated to the patch and matrix striatal compartments. Retrograde axonal tracing that fills the dendrites of these projection neurons, intracellular filling of individual neurons and Golgi impregnation studies have shown that the dendrites of medium spiny neurons remain confined for the most part to the compartment in which the cell body is located (*2, 9, 10, 19*). Thus inputs to the striatal patches target patch projection neurons and inputs to the matrix projection neurons. Patch and matrix neurons themelves have distinct targets in the substantia nigra (*9, 10, 12*). Striatal patch neurons provide inputs to the location of the cell bodies of dopaminergic neurons that are located in the ventral tier of the substantia nigra pars compacta and to the islands of dopaminergic neurons located in the pars reticulata. On the other hand, striatal matrix neurons provide inputs to the parts of the substantia nigra pars reticulata in which are located the GABAergic nigrothalamic and nigrotectal neurons. The dendrites of some dopaminergic neurons extend into the pars reticulata region receiving matrix inputs. The function of these dopaminergic dendrites is unclear, as it is suggested that they may themselves release dopamine. The compartmental segregation of the dendritic arbors of medium spiny neurons, and their distinct projections to different subdivisions of the substantia nigra, suggest that this organization provides parallel but segregated input-output pathways through the striatum.

Patch and matrix neurons share many of the same neurochemicals. It is still a matter of some controversy what percentage of the medium spiny neurons utilize GABA as their transmitter, some suggesting nearly all and some suggesting roughly half that number. Regardless, both patch and matrix neurons appear to contain GABA. Different subpopulations of striatal neurons express the peptides enkephalin, substance P and dynorphin (*15*). Since roughly

50–60% of the medium spiny neurons express each of these peptides there is a considerable overlap amongst populations coexpressing more than one peptide. However, there appears to be a relatively even distribution of each of these peptide-expressing neurons in both patch and matrix compartments. One neurochemical that has been demonstrated to be preferentially expressed by only matrix and not patch neurons is the calcium binding protein, calbindin D_{28kD}, (CaBP) (*12*). This protein provides a reliable marker of the compartmental organization of the striatum. Moreover, the distribution of CaBP immunoreactive terminals in the substantia nigra arising specifically from matrix neurons as opposed to the distribution of substance P immunoreactive terminals in the substantia nigra arising

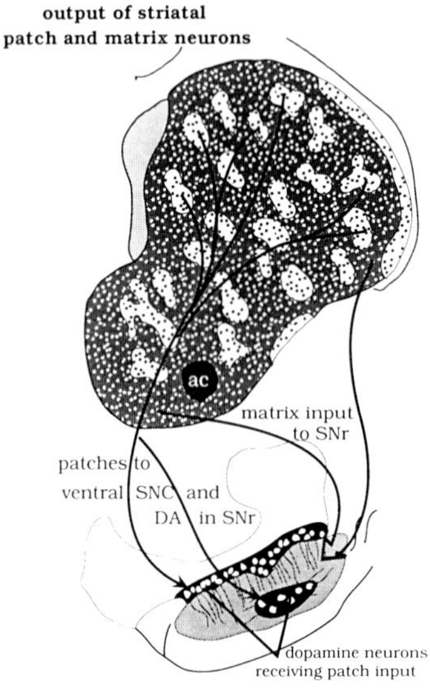

Fig. 1. A schematic drawing of coronal sections through the striatum (top) and substantia nigra (bottom) shows the compartmental organization of striatonigral projections. Neurons located in the striatal patches project to the location of the cell bodies of dopaminergic neurons located in the ventral tier of the substantia nigra pars compacta and to the islands of dopaminergic cells in the substantia nigra pars reticulata. Neurons located in the striatal matrix project to the non-dopaminergic regions of the substantia nigra pars reticulata. In this region are located the GABAergic nigral cells that project to the thalamus, superior colliculus and pedunculopontine nucleus. Also, the dendrites of the dopaminergic neurons that are the targets of the patch projection system extend into the region receiving matrix inputs. The matrix projection neurons and their terminals express CaBP.

from both compartments, confirms the differences in the nigral targets of matrix and patch neurons.

II. COMPARTMENTAL ORGANIZATION OF MESOSTRIATAL SYSTEMS

Neurons in the ventral midbrain areas, which include the ventral tegmental area, substantia nigra and retrorubral area, provide a major feedback system to the striatum. Between 85–90% of these neurons are dopaminergic. Using the *Phaseolus vulgaris*-leucoagglutinin (PHA-L) anterograde axonal tract tracing method (*8*) combined with co-localization of immunoreactivity for tyrosine hydroxylase to distinguish dopaminergic from non-dopaminergic PHA-L labeled mesostriatal fibers, three mesostriatal afferent systems have been identified (*13*). These systems are distinct in the morphology of their fibers, in their distribution to the patch and matrix striatal compartments, in their distribution in the midbrain, and in their neurochemical phenotype. One mesostriatal system is non-dopaminergic and arises from neurons in the substantia nigra pars reticulata. These neurons constitute approximately 15% of the neurons in the ventral midbrain that project to the striatum, as determined by combined retrograde axonal transport and immunohistochemical localization of tyrosine hydroxylase. The morphology of the projection fibers of these neurons is distinct from the dopaminergic striatal afferents, as determined by combining PHA-L labeling of nigrostriatal afferents and tyrosine hydroxylase immunoreactivity. PHA-L labeled nigrostriatal afferents that are non-dopaminergic are characterized by their relatively thick fibers (0.5–1 μm) with large bulbous boutons (up to 2 μm in diameter). These afferents are distributed selectively in the striatal matrix compartment. The other two mesostriatal afferent systems are dopaminergic. Both of these systems are characterized by relatively fine caliber fibers with boutons that are only slightly larger than the fibers themselves. The two dopaminergic systems are distinguished on the basis of their differential projections to the striatal patch and matrix compartments. Matrix-directed afferents arise from neurons in the ventral tegmental area, dorsal tier of the substantia nigra pars compacta and retrorubral area, whereas patch-directed afferents arise from neurons in the ventral tier of the substantia nigra pars compacta and from dopaminergic neurons in the substantia nigra pars reticulata. Thus, matrix and patch directed mesostriatal afferents arise from dorsal and ventral sets of neurons.

There are several other characteristics that distinguish the dorsal matrix-directed and ventral patch-directed dopaminergic neurons. 1) The dendrites of the matrix directed neurons extend in domains within the area of the dorsal set of dopaminergic neurons, whereas the dendrites of patch-directed neurons extend into the non-dopaminergic area of the substantia nigra pars reticulata. This point is noteworthy because there is some evidence that dopaminergic neuron dendrites may release dopamine, possibly for the purpose of autoregulation. Also, in thc casc of thc vcntral, patch-directed neurons, the cell bodies of these neurons appear to receive inputs specifically from the striatal patch compartment, whereas the area into which their dendrites extend, pars reticulata, is in the area that receives inputs from the striatal matrix. It is therefore possible that regulation of inputs to the cell bodies and dendrites of these neurons is controlled by different striatal output systems. The dorsal matrix-directed dopaminergic neurons do not appear to receive a major input from either striatal compartment. 2) The two mesostriatal dopaminergic systems are also different biochemically. The dorsal matrix-directed dopaminergic neurons express a specific CaBP (*14*). This protein is also expressed in the output neurons of the striatal matrix, which specifically project to the substantia nigra pars reticulata (*12*). The ventral patch-directed dopaminergic neurons do not express this protein. 3) The two mesostriatal dopaminergic systems develop asynchronously. In rats at birth the dopaminergic system to the patches appears to be in place, whereas the input to the matrix has not yet fully developed. Specific lesions of the patch dopaminergic system, made by injecting the toxin 6-hydroxydopamine into the striatum at birth, result in a persistent and specific deafferentation of the patches. Such a treatment has a lesser effect on the later developing matrix system, and results in the adult in the maintenance of the dorsal matrix-directed (CaBP positive) neurons, and absence of the ventral patch-directed neurons (*14*).

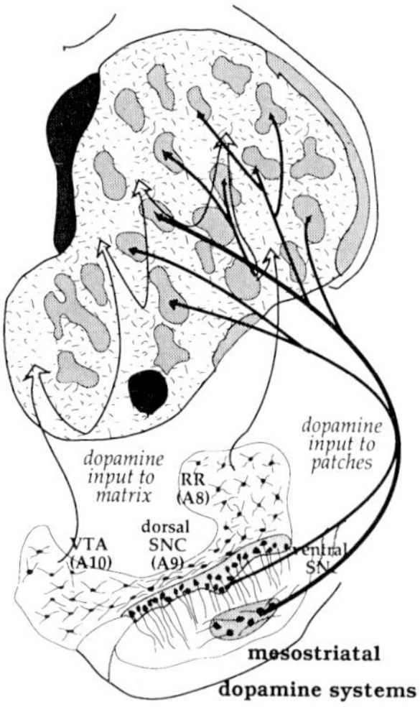

Fig. 2. Diagram of the compartmental organization of the dopaminergic mesostriatal systems. Dopaminergic afferents to the striatal matrix arise from a dorsal set of neurons that are located in the ventral tegmental area (VTA/A10 cell group), dorsal tier of the substantia nigra pars compacta (dorsal SNc/A9 cell group) and retrorubral area (RR/A8 cell group). These neurons also express CaBP. Dopaminergic afferents to the striatal patches arise from a ventral set of neurons that are located in the ventral tier of the substantia nigra pars compacta (ventral SNc/A9 cell group) and from islands of dopaminergic neurons in the substantia nigra pars reticulata.

III. COMPARTMENTAL ORGANIZATION OF CORTICO-STRIATAL SYSTEMS

The compartmental organization of the corticostriatal projection was examined with PHA-L anterograde axonal tracer. Injections of PHA-L were made to label cortical projections of frontal lobe areas in the rat including the infralimbic, prelimbic, anterior cingulate, medial agranular motor, and lateral agranular motor cortices. Each cortical area injected is shown to provide inputs to both compartments, with restricted inputs to the patch and matrix compartments being related to the laminar origin of the corticostriatal projection. Deep layer V and layer VI corticostriatal neurons project to the patches, whereas superficial layer V and supragranular corticostriatal neurons project to the matrix. Additionally, injections that label patch-directed inputs also label crossed corticocortical projections that are restricted to deep layer V and layer VI. Conversely, injections that label matrix-directed inputs label inputs to more superficial layers of the contralateral cortex. The relative contribution of patch and matrix corticostriatal projections varies amongst the cortical areas examined such that infralimbic and prelimbic cortical areas provide a greater number of inputs to the patches than to the matrix, whereas the reverse obtains for the cingulate and agranular motor cortices.

These findings demonstrate that the compartmental organization of corticostriatal inputs from the frontal pole of the rat are related to the laminar origin of the projection neurons and secondarily to the cytoarchitectonic area of origin. Previous studies have suggested that the compartmental organization of corticostriatal inputs is dependent on the cortical area of origin. Most compelling in this regard is the finding that the prelimbic cortex, which had previously been reported to project selectively to the patch compartment, projects to both compartments (*6*, *9*). Projections to the patch and matrix compartments from the prelimbic cortex area are related to the laminar origin of the corticostriatal projection neurons in that PHA-L labeled afferents that are restricted to the patches result from injections that label mostly deep layer V neurons and crossed inputs to the deeper layers of the homotypic cortex, whereas labeled afferents that are restricted to the matrix result from injections of more superficial prelimbic cortical layers and also crossed inputs to more superficial layers of the homotypic cortex. This laminar pattern of corticostriatal organization is not unique to the prelimbic cortex, but is also observed with injections into the cingulate, medial and lateral agranular motor cortices. There does appear to be a differential density of patch *versus* matrix corticostriatal projections from different cortical areas, such that inputs to the patches are denser from the prelimbic cortex than from the motor cortices. This is consistent with retrograde labeling studies of corticostriatal neurons, which report a greater number of deeper layer corticostriatal neurons in the prelimbic cortex than the motor cortices (*7*, *27*).

In attempting to determine the functional significance of the striatal compartments it may be advantageous to relate this organization to analogous organizations in other systems. The cerebral cortex displays a number of heterogenous organizational schemes (see ref.

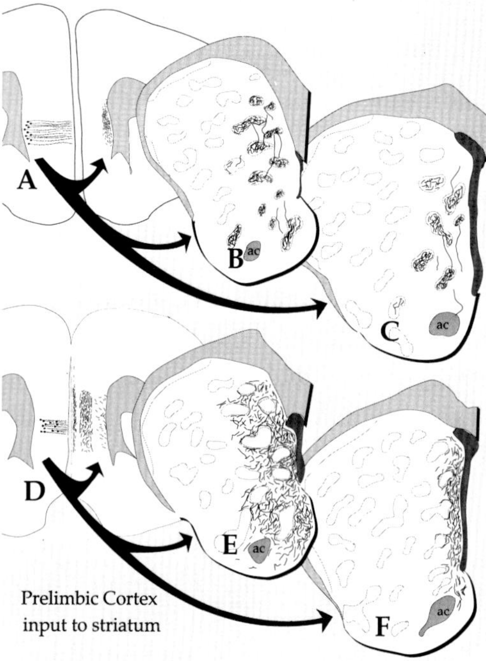

Fig. 3. Schematic of PHA-L labeling demonstrating laminar origin of corticostriatal inputs to the patch and matrix compartments from the prelimbic cortex of the rat. In A, PHA-L labeled neurons are located in layer VI and deep layer V and provide crossed inputs to the deep layers of the homotypic cortex. This injection labels inputs directed to the striatal patch compartment (B and C). In D, PHA-L labeled neurons are located in more superficial parts of layer V and in supragranular layers and provide crossed inputs to the superficial layers of the homotypic cortex. This injection labels inputs directed to the striatal matrix compartment (E and F).

21 for review). First, the cortex is a highly laminated structure. Second, the cortex may be subdivided on the basis of differences in laminar thickness that establish specific cytoarchitecturally defined areas. Third, these areas may be further subdivided on the basis of a columnar organization, which is related to, among other things, the afferent and efferent connections, and certain neurohistochemical markers. While the present study provides the strongest suggestion that the striatal compartments are related to the laminar organization of the cortex it is consistent with other findings as well. From a development point of view a case may be made for the analogous generation of cortical laminae and striatal compartments. Neurons in both structures are generated in a proliferative zone and migrate along radial glia to obtain their final position. In the cortex, neurons that generate the different laminae are born at roughly the same time, and similarly in the striatum there are two major waves of cell births that generate the patch and matrix compartments (*26*). Notably, both the patch neurons and the deeper cortical laminar neurons are born prior to the matrix and more superficially located cortical neurons. There are regional differences in the cell birth dates in both the cortex and striatum, but these appear to be secondary to the generation of the laminae in the cortex and the compartments in the striatum. From an evolutionary point of view there also seems to be evidence to support this idea. A comparison of the number and size of columns in the cortex in primates suggests that progression in evolution is marked by an increase in the number but not the size of cortical columns (*3*). A similar comparison of the striatal patches suggests a different evolutionary progression, with an increase in the size but not the number of patches. This is not to say that there is no relationship between either the cytoarchitectural or columnar organization of the cortex and striatal compartmentation. As mentioned, there are differences in the number of patch-projecting neurons compared with matrix-projecting neurons among different cortical areas.

Heterogeneity in the striatum demonstrated by the distribution of neurochemical markers and the input, output and intrinsic connections of the striatum has generated substantial interest in how this compartmental organization is related to the function of the basal ganglia. Nauta *et al.* introduced the concept that the striatum was a site at which motor and limbic functions are integrated (*24*). This view was based on the neuroanatomical findings that the ventral striatum, which receives inputs from limbic structures such as the amygdala and hippocampus, provides inputs to the dopaminergic cells in the midbrain that provide a major feedback system to the dorsal (or motor) regions of the striatum. Our findings that inputs to the dopaminergic nigrostriatal feedback system arise not strictly from the ventral striatum but from the patches distributed in both the ventral and dorsal striatum, suggest that the patches may serve a function similar to that ascribed to the ventral striatum. This is reinforced by findings that the amygdala and the prelimbic cortex, which receives a major input from the amygdala, project to the striatal patches. The present findings that both the prelimbic cortex and motor cortices project to both compartments suggest a need for reassessing the idea that the patches are strictly related to the limbic system. An alternative scheme is proposed that relates the compartmental organization of the striatum to the differential linkage of phylogenetically older connections with the patches and phylogenetically newer connections with the matrix. This scheme is intended to take into account the existence of phylogenetically older connections in neocortical areas. An analogous organization has been proposed for the laminar organization of corticocortical connections in primates (*1*). A generalized scheme has been suggested in which within any given cortical area there is a progression of afferents arising from supragranular to infragranular laminae that veries according to cytoarchiectonic differentiation, which is related to the phylogeny, of the areas that are the source of these afferents. Thus the present findings that point to a relationship between the striatal compartments and the laminar organization of the cortex suggest that, rather than attempting to ascribe "limbic" *versus* "non-limbic" functions to the striatal compartments, a more cogent strategy is to relate the functional significance of the compartments to common determinants of their connections with other brain systems.

SUMMARY

A major system through which the cerebral cortex affects behavior is by way of connections with the basal ganglia. Our studies have examined the major component of the basal ganglia, the striatum, to show how the relationships between extrinsic connections (*i.e.*, corticostriatal input and striatonigral output systems) and intrinsic striatal architecture relate to functional organization. Neuroanatomical techniques have shown that the striatum is composed of two distinct compartments: the *patches* and *matrix*. Over 95% of the neurons of the striatum are medium spiny projection neurons, which provide the major output of this nucleus. The segregation of separate populations of patch and matrix neurons, whose dendrites remain confined to their respective compartment, forms a morphologic basis of the striatal compartmentation. Targets of the outputs of these compartments are distinct; patch neurons project to the location of dopaminergic neurons in the substantia nigra, whereas matrix neurons project to the GABAergic neurons in the substantia nigra pars reticulata. Moreover, while both patch and matrix neurons share many phenotypic features, including common morphology and common neurotransmitter/peptides, they differ in the select expression of a CaBP by the matrix projection neurons. Afferent inputs to the striatum are also compartmentalized. The dopaminergic feedback projection system from the midbrain is also compartmentalized. Two separate mesostriatal systems have been identified. Matrix-directed afferents originate from a dorsal set of neurons, including dopaminergic neurons in the ventral tegmental area, dorsal tier of the substantia nigra pars compacta and retrorubral area. Patch-directed afferents originate from dopaminergic neurons in the ventral tier of the pars compacta and from dopaminergic neurons located in the pars reticulata, both of which extend dendrites into the pars reticulata. Moreover, matrix-directed mesostriatal dopaminergic afferents also express CaBP, whereas patch-directed neurons do not. Corticostriatal inputs respect the compartmental boundaries with the following organization: deeper layer V corticostriatal neurons project to the patches, whereas more superficial layer V and supragranular corticostriatal neurons project to the matrix. The relative density of patch *versus* matrix projecting corticostriatal neurons varies among cortical areas, with neocortical areas possessing more of the latter. These neuroanatomical studies suggest that the striatal patch and matrix compartments constitute separate and parallel input-output pathways. The compartmental organization of the corticostriatal system suggests further a functional analogy between the striatal compartments and the laminar organization of the cortex.

REFERENCES

1 Barbas, H. (1986). *J. Comp. Neurol.* **244**, 492-510.
2 Bolam, J.P., Izzo, I.N., and Graybiel, A.M. (1988). *Neuroscience* **24**, 853-875.
3 Bugbee, N.M. and Goldman-Rakic, P.S. (1983). *J. Comp. Neurol.* **220**, 355-364.
4 Deniau, J.M., Feger, J., and LeGuyader. C. (1976). *Brain Res.* **104**, 152-156.
5 Deniau, J.M., Chevalier, G., and Feger, J. (1978). *Neurosci. Lett.* **10**, 215-220.
6 Donoghue, J.P. and Herkenham, M. (1986). *Brain Res.* **365**, 397-403.
7 Ferino, F., Thierry, A.M., Saffroy, M., and Glowinski, J. (1987) *Brain Res.* **417**, 257-266.
8 Gerfen, C.R. and Sawchenko, P.E. (1984) *Brain Res.* **290**, 219-238.
9 Gerfen, C.R. (1984). *Nature* **311**, 461-464.
10 Gerfen, C.R. (1985). *J. Comp. Neurol.* **236**, 454-476.
11 Gerfen, C.R. (1988). *J. Elec. Micro. Tech.* **10**, 247-281.
12 Gerfen, C.R., Baimbridge, K.G., and Miller, J.J. (1985) *Proc. Natl. Acad. Sci. U.S.A.* **82**, 8780-8784.
13 Gerfen, C.R., Herkenham, M., and Thibault, J. (1987). *J. Neurosci.* **7**, 3915-3934.
14 Gerfen, C.R., Baimbridge, K.G., and Thibault, J. (1987). *J. Neurosci.* **7**, 3935-3944.
15 Gerfen, C.R. and Young, W.S. III (1988). *Brain Res.* **460**, 161-167.
16 Graybiel, A.M. and Ragsdale, C.W. Jr. (1978). *Proc. Natl. Acad. Sci. U.S.A.* **75**, 5723-5726.
17 Grofova, I. (1975). *Brain Res.* **91**, 286-291.
18 Herkenham, M. and Pert, C.B. (1981). *Nature* **291**, 415-418.
19 Herkenham, M., Moon Edley, S., and Stuart, J. (1984). *Neuroscience* **11**, 561-593.
20 Hikosaka, O. and Wurtz, R.H. (1983). *J. Neurophysiol.* **49**, 1268-1284.
21 Jones, E.G. (1984). In *Cerebral Cortex*, vol. 1, ed. Peters, A. and Jones, E.G., pp. 521-533. New York: Plenum Press.
22 Kemp, J.M. and Powell, T.P.S. (1971). *Phil. Trans. R. Soc. Lond. (Biol.)* **262**, 383-401.
23 Kitai, S.T., Koscis, J.D., Preston, R.J., and Sugimori, M. (1976). *Brain Res.* **109**, 601-606.
24 Nauta, W.J.H., Smith, G.P., Faull, R.L.M., and Domesick, V.B. (1978). *Neuroscience* **3**, 385-401.
25 Pert, C.B., Kuhar, M.J., and Snyder, S.H. (1976). *Proc. Natl. Acad. Sci. U.S.A.* **73**, 3729-3733.
26 van der Kooy, D. and Fishell, G. (1987). *Brain Res.* **401**, 155-161.
27 Wilson, C.J. (1987). *J. Comp. Neurol.* **263**, 567-580.
28 Wilson, C.J. and Groves, P.M. (1980). *J. Comp. Neurol.* **194**, 599-615.

8
MOTOR REGULATION IN THE BASAL GANGLIA

MINORU KIMURA

Department of Physiology, Jichi Medical School, Minamikawachi-machi, Tochigi 329-04, Japan

Although it has been suggested that the basal ganglia have a motor function, primarily based on the unique movement disorders observed in patients with basal ganglia damage (*8*, *20*), the role of the basal ganglia in motor control is still not clear. Recent anatomical and physiological studies have elicited several important clues regarding the mechanism of operation of the basal ganglia in movement and cognitive functions. This paper provides a review of our recent neurophysiological research on the putamen and the globus pallidus and considers the ways of operation of the basal ganglia in voluntary movement. The paper will describe the neuronal activity of the putamen and globus pallidus of the monkey during learned arm movement. Functional classes of putamen neurons and the signal content in these neuronal activities will be reviewed. Next, the neuronal information transferred from the putamen to the globus pallidus in performance of learned movement will be described. Finally, based on observations which show that sensory responses and movement-locked activities of basal ganglia neurons are strongly dependent on the circumstances in which an external stimulus is presented and movement is performed, the argument will be made that the basal ganglia may be involved in the selection of an appropriate movement through associating a particular learned movement with a contextual cue derived from either the environment or internal memory storage.

I. NEURONAL RELATION OF THE PUTAMEN TO LEARNED MOVEMENT

Recent anatomical (*14, 18*) and physiological (*2, 5*) experiments have revealed that the primate putamen is zonally organized with rostrocaudally elongated bands of different somatotopy which are determined through the corticostriatal projections from the sensory-motor areas. We have attempted to identify the optimum condition to activate cells in the basal ganglia in order to know the signal content in the activity of basal ganglia neurons during learned arm movements. Neuronal activity was recorded in the putamen and globus pallidus during two behavioral tasks: 1) the arm movement (AM) task, which is a visually triggered repetitive (3 times) flexion-extension of an elbow joint across a target; and 2) the no movement (NM) task, which is visual attention to the sensory trigger stimulus identical to that used in the AM task but without initiating any arm movement.

Two categories of neurons have been found in the monkey striatum. The type I neuron exhibits tonic spontaneous discharges at about 2–7 Hz but does not exhibit burst discharges in relation to any behavioral event, while the type II neuron shows very low spontaneous discharges but exhibits burst discharges in relation to a sensory event and/or learned movements (*2, 6, 15, 16*).

Figure 1 shows the activity of a type I cell. Interspike interval analysis shows that most spikes occur at intervals between 100 msec and 200 msec (average, 153 msec) when the monkey is at rest (Fig. 1B). The type I cell yields responses to an external event. In the AM task, the visual stimulus calling for a sequence of repetitive arm movements from a point of extension (T_{ex}) evoked a pause in the tonic discharges with a latency of about 150 msec, while the solenoid click to indicate the delivery of reward juice (R) after the completion of the repetitive arm movements evoked excitation with a 90 msec latency. The tonic activity was not modulated during either arm

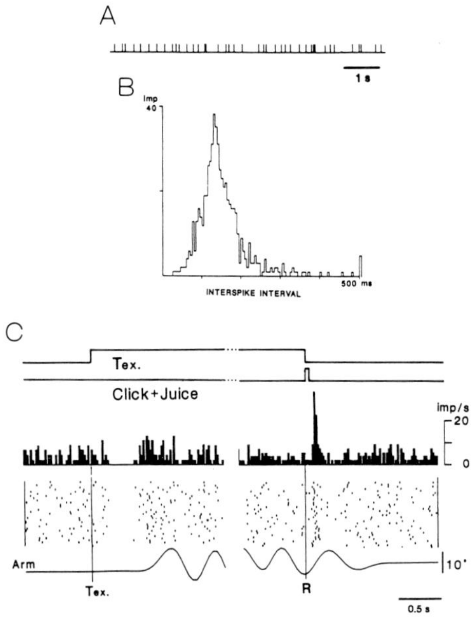

Fig. 1. Activity of a type I cell in the putamen. A: pen-recorded tonic discharges of the cell. B: interspike interval histogram of the cell, calculated while the monkey was at rest. An average spike interval was 153 msec. A minimal number of spikes occurred at intervals of less than 50 msec. C: the raster and response histogram of the cell to the learned sensory trigger stimulus. The type I cell showed inhibition of tonic discharges to the light stimulus calling for repetitive arm movements from extension (T_{ex}), and a short latency excitation by the click of a solenoid valve (R).

movements or orofacial movements used to consume the reward (Fig. 1C). The important characteristic of the responses to the external event is that the identical stimulus does not evoke responses when the stimulus is presented independently of the learned behavior, and thus the stimulus does not trigger the learned movement. This indicated that the response was not a simple sensory response.

A group of type II cells showed phasic burst discharges in response to the external stimulus. Most of the type II cell responses appeared when the stimulus was used by the monkey as a trigger for the learned movement similarly to type I cell. The responses were, however, strongly enhanced when the monkey indicated anticipation of the event beforehand, and they were almost completely depressed when the same event occurred independently of the behavioral context. On the other hand, about one-fifth of the responses of both type I and type II cells occurred independently of the behavioral context.

In the central sector of the rostrocaudally elongated bands of the putamen, many cells showed phasic discharges in relation to arm movements. Microstimulation through a recording electrode in this area evoked discrete movements of the wrist, forearm or upper arm with a low stimulus current, thus the arm area could be defined in the putamen through microstimulation effects (*1*, *15*). Two categories of movement-related cells were classified in the putamen, type IIa and type IIb cells. Figure 2A, B illustrates the activity of a type IIa cell recorded in the "arm area". The cell showed phasic burst discharges once before a sequence of the visually triggered repetitive arm movements, but during the second and the third movements, the cell was almost inactive, although the movement parameters such as amplitude and velocity of repetitive movements did not differ significantly (Fig. 2A). The raster display of impulse discharges was reordered according to the reaction time of the first flexion after the visual trigger (T_{fx}) and the movement onset was marked on each raster. The phasic discharges occurred with a fairly constant latency of 110 msec after the visual trigger and ceased as soon as the first flexion of the arm was initiated. The task was switched from AM to NM where the visual trigger was presented while the monkey's arm was mechanically restricted; reward juice was delivered 1 sec after the visual stimulus. The monkey's attempts to initiate the learned arm movement against the restrictive device were soon abandoned. The type IIa cell showed burst discharges at the first trial when the monkey exhibited an intention to move (raster with arrow in Fig. 2B), but thereafter showed only a few spikes in succeeding trials where no intention to move was shown. Thus, the phasic discharges with a fairly short latency after a visual trigger (100–150 msec) and the presence of visually triggered activity without movement indicated that the type IIa cell response is composed of visual stimulus-related as well as movement-related components, or "visuomovement" properties, although they cannot always be distinguished by time sequences.

In strong contrast to the type IIa cells, the type IIb cells showed

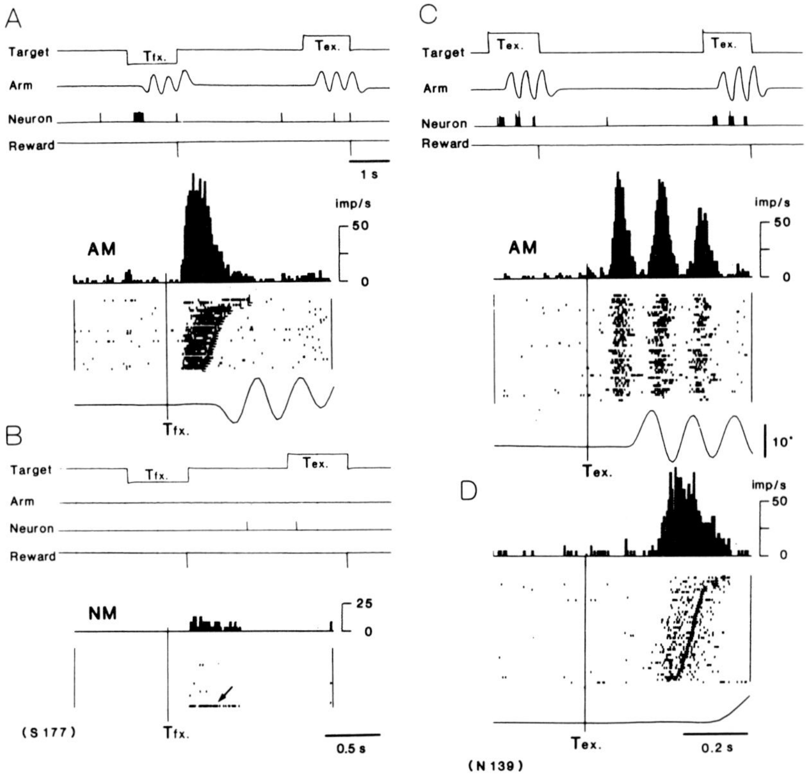

Fig. 2. Activity of two categories of type II cells during learned arm movements. Records A and B were obtained from a type IIa cell. Rasters of impulse discharges in A are reordered based on the reaction time of the arm movement after the presentation of the target light (T_{fx}), and the 'L' on each raster line marks the movement onset. Rasters of impulse discharges during NM task in B are arranged in chronological order from bottom to top, and the first trial after switching the task from AM to NM is indicated by an arrow. C, D: activity of a type IIb cell. The rasters of impulse discharges in D are reordered according to the reaction time and movement onsets are marked by asterisks. Time scale in B applies to A, B, and C, while the scale in D applies only to D (modified from Kimura. (*15*)).

burst discharges which were time-locked to each repetitive arm movement, as illustrated in Fig. 2C. This pattern of activity was identical to that of the prime mover muscles. The burst activity was more closely time-locked to the movement onset than to the visual trigger (Fig. 2D).

The onset times of burst discharges in type IIa cells preceded those of EMGs in the prime mover muscles by about 100 msec, while most of the type IIb cells were activated after the prime mover EMGs had appeared.

It is unlikely that type IIa cells are engaged unconditionally in control of supporting muscles for the elbow flexion-extensions in the AM task for the following reasons. First, microstimulation at the recording site of type IIa cells evoked discrete activation of the wrist and arm muscles. Second, about 30% of the type IIa cells were activated by passive manipulation of the elbow and wrist joint. Third, the type IIa cells showed not only movement-locked activity but also trigger stimulus-dependent activity (Fig. 2A, B).

II. THE INFORMATION TRANSFERRED FROM THE PUTAMEN TO THE GLOBUS PALLIDUS

In order to determine what neural information is transferred from the putamen to the globus pallidus during voluntary limb movement, a microelectrode was introduced into the globus pallidus to deliver a stimulus current while the unit activity was recorded in the putamen through another electrode (*17*). After identifying the cell type (type I, IIa, or IIb) based on the discharge characteristics of the putamen cell during the behavioral tasks, examination was carried out to determine if the recorded cell was activated antidromically through electrical stimulation of the globus pallidus.

Out of 32 thus identified cells projecting to the globus pallidus, 10 were type IIa, and 13 were type IIb cells; all of these cells exhibited phasic discharges time-locked to the movement. The remaining 9 cells were either type IIa or type IIb. They were not type I, since they did not show tonic spontaneous discharges characteristic of the type I cells. In more than 40 cells tested, no type I cell was identified as projecting to the globus pallidus. Thus, it was revealed that the type IIa and type IIb cell activities which have a movement-related component were transferred to the globus pallidus, while neither the type I cells nor the type II cells responding to an external event seemed to be a projection cell.

The research of Delong (*7*), and that of Mitchell, Richardson, and Delong (*21*) demonstrated that neurons in the globus pallidus showed phasic modulation of their high frequency discharges in relation to a learned arm movement. Kimura, Rajkowski, and Evarts demonstrated that globus pallidus cells showed a decrement of high frequency discharges with a short constant latency after the sensory trigger stimulus for repetitive body movements (*16*). These cell activities had a similar profile to those of type I and type IIa putamen cells, since the activity was almost completely depressed when the stimulus was presented independently of the behavioral context.

III. FUNCTIONAL CONSIDERATION OF PUTAMINOPALLIDAL SYSTEM

The most striking features of neuronal activity in the putamen and globus pallidus are behavioral enhancement of the responses to external events and dependence of movement-locked activity on whether the movement occurs as an initial or succeeding movement of a sequence of movements (*15, 16*). Similar behavioral enhancement of sensory responses has been recently reported in relation to the learned eye movement task in cells of the caudate nucleus and the substantia nigra pars reticulata (*10–12*).

The enhanced sensory responses of the putamen cells are similar to those observed in the posterior parietal cortex. In the cortex, the enhancement of responses in many cells occurred in association with the visual stimulus calling for not only eye, but also hand movements, but did not occur when the learned movement was not triggered (*4*). The cells in the supplementary motor area were reported to respond to visual and auditory stimuli (*23, 24*). Most of them were dependent upon the triggering context of the sensory stimuli. Thus, the remarkable modulation of sensory activity and the dependency of movement-related activity on the triggered context in the putamen and globus pallidus cells leads to the following point of view on the function of the basal ganglia: one of the essential operations of the putaminopallidal system is to select an appropriate movement by associating a particular learned movement with the contextual cues derived from the external environment, but the system is less related to detailed parameterization of movement. This operation would contribute mostly to the initiation of a learned movement, but it does not necessarily exclude contributions to movement execution. In fact, the activities of type IIb cells would contribute to the execution process of movement, which is consistent with the suggestions noted in previous studies (*6, 8, 19*).

It has been suggested that most efferent activities from the internal segment of the globus pallidus are transmitted to the cortical motor areas, particularly to the supplementary motor and then to the primary motor area through the pallidothalamocortical loop (*22*). In addition, it is stated that a part of these would directly descend to the spinal cord through the tectospinal or reticulospinal path (*8, 9*). This scheme of neuronal connections indicates the temporal aspect of neuronal activity. Although the type IIa cell activity occurs about 100 msec before EMGs of prime mover muscles on average, it may not be early enough to drive the initial part of the prime mover muscle activity by itself. However, movement-related as well as sensory-related activities in the putamen could increase the excitability of cortical cells and enhance the effect of converging movement-related inputs from other brain areas such as the cerebellum, as suggested electrophysiologically (*13*). Anatomical and electrophysiological data on such a convergence showed negative results at the level of the thalamus and the premotor, supplementary motor cortex (*22, 25, 26*), but such convergence was observed in the primary motor cortex (*13*). Recently, convergence from the basal ganglia and the cerebellum on a small number of cells in the VA-VL nuclear complex of the thalamus was observed (*13*), and the modulation of cerebellothalamocortical transmission correlating with changes of the discharge rate of substantia nigra cells was demonstrated in the rat (*3*).

It has been demonstrated that the basal ganglia output from the substantia nigra pars reticulata exerts strong inhibitory action on the cells in the intermediate layer of the superior colliculus, and that the activity of the nigral cells related to saccadic eye movements has a disinhibitory effect on the collicular cells (*12*). It is not clear at present whether disinhibitory processes are also involved in the operation of the pallidothalamocortical system. However, the cells in the internal segment of the globus pallidus showed not only a decrease but also an increase of high frequency discharges in relation to limb movements (*21*, unpublished observation), while the cells in the substantia nigra pars reticulata showed only a decrease of discharges in relation to an eye movement task (*11, 12*).

Acknowledgments
I would like to thank Prof. Kyoji Maekawa for his encouragement and Ms. Midori Okada for her technical assistance. This work was supported by a grant (#63570063) and a Grant-in-Aid for Scientific Research on Priority Areas from the Japanese Ministry of Education, Science and Culture.

REFERENCES

1 Alexander, G.E. and DeLong, M.R. (1985). *J. Neurophysiol.* **53**, 1401–1416.
2 Alexander, G.E. and DeLong, M.R. (1985). *J. Neurophysiol.* **53**, 1417–1430.
3 Buee, J., Deniau, J.M., and Chevalier, G. (1986). *Exp. Brain Res.* **65**, 241–244.
4 Bushnell, M.C., Goldberg, M.E., and Robinson, D.L. (1981). *J. Neurophysiol.* **46**, 755–771.
5 Crutcher, M.D. and DeLong, M.R. (1984). *Exp. Brain Res.* **53**, 233–243.
6 Crutcher, M.D. and DeLong, M.R. (1984). *Exp. Brain Res.* **53**, 244–258.
7 DeLong, M.R. (1971). *J. Neurophysiol.* **34**, 414–427.
8 DeLong, M.R. and Georgopoulos, A.P. (1981). In *Handbook of Physiology*, ed. Brookhart *et al.*, pp. 1017–1061. Bethesda, MD: American Physiological Society.
9 Graybiel, A.M. and Ragsdale, C.W. (1979). In *Development and Chemical Specificity of Neurons*, ed. Quenod, M., Kreutzberg, G.W., and Bloom, F.E., pp. 239–283. Amsterdam: Elsevier.
10 Hikosaka, O. and Sakamoto, M. (1986). *Exp. Brain Res.* **63**, 659–662.
11 Hikosaka, O. and Wurtz, R.H. (1983). *J. Neurophysiol.* **49**, 1230–1253.
12 Hikosaka, O. and Wurtz, R.H. (1983). *J. Neurophysiol.* **49**, 1285–1301.
13 Jinnai, K., Nambu, A., and Yoshida, S. (1987). *Exp. Brain Res.* **69**, 67–76.
14 Jones, E.G., Coulter, J.D., Burton, T., and Porter, R. (1977). *J. Comp. Neurol.* **173**, 53–80.
15 Kimura, M. (1986). *Neurosci. Res.* **3**, 436–443.
16 Kimura, M., Rajkowski, J., and Evarts, E.V. (1984). *Proc. Natl. Acad. Sci. U.S.A.* **81**, 4998-5001.
17 Kimura, M., Shimazaki, H., and Kato, M. (1987). *Neurosci. Res.* (Suppl.) **5**, S30.
18 Künzle, H. (1975). *Brain Res.* **88**, 195–209.
19 Liles, S.L. (1985). *J. Neurophysiol.* **53**, 217–236.
20 Marsden, C.D. (1982). *Neurology* **32**, 514–538.
21 Mitchell, S.J., Richardson, F.H., and DeLong, M.R. (1987). *Exp. Brain Res.* **68**, 491–505.
22 Schell, G.R. and Strick, P.L. (1984). *J. Neurosci.* **4**, 539–560.

23 Tanji, J., Taniguchi, K., and Saga, T. (1980). *J. Neurophysiol.* **43**, 60–68.
24 Tanji, J. and Kurata, K. (1985). *J. Neurophysiol.* **53**, 129–141.
25 Uno, M., Yoshida, M., and Hirota, I. (1970). *Exp. Brain Res.* **10**, 121–139.
26 Yamamoto, T., Hassler, R., Huber, C., Wagner, A., and Sasaki, K. (1983). *Exp. Brain Res.* **51**, 77–87.

9

MOTOR PROGRAMMING IN BASAL GANGLIA

OKIHIDE HIKOSAKA

National Institute for Physiological Sciences, Okazaki, Aichi 444, Japan

The concept that the basal ganglia have motor functions has been derived mainly from clinical observations. A variety of motor diseases are caused by malfunction of the basal ganglia. Eye movement can also be affected. The study of eye movement offers several opportunities to observe the function of higher motor structures, including the basal ganglia. Ocular muscles are much simpler than limb muscles and, accordingly, eye movements are simpler than limb movements. Furthermore, or because of this, the brainstem neural mechanism underlying eye movements has been thoroughly delineated (*15*); even computer simulation models have been successfully adopted (*13*). I find this background to be of great advantage in searching for the trace of motor programs in the higher motor areas. The basal ganglia is in a strategic position.

In the first part of this paper, I will summarize the hardware of the basal ganglia involved in the initiation of saccadic eye movements. Secondly, I will consider the functional role of the basal ganglia in comparison with other motor areas. Finally, I will provide some speculative thoughts on the role of the basal ganglia in the execution of motor programming.

I. BASAL GANGLIA INITIATE MOVEMENTS BY DISINHIBITION

Eye movement-related signals have been found in the caudate nucleus and the substantia nigra pars reticulata (SNr). First, I must emphasize the difference between these two areas. The caudate nucleus is an extremely quiet area. The background discharge rates of caudate neurons are usually lower than 1 spike/sec. By contrast, the SNr is a very busy area: the mean background discharge rates are usually between 50 and 100 spikes/sec. The discharge varies minimally with the levels of wakefulness. Such a big difference in background activity points to a basic mode of basal ganglia operation, which will become clear if we look at single cell activities in relation to saccadic eye movements.

Hikosaka and Wurtz (*4–6*) studied the spike activity of SNr neurons in rhesus monkeys in relation to their eye movements. The monkey sat in a primate chair with his head fixed. Eye movements were recorded using the search coil technique. Interestingly, SNr neurons scarcely changed their spike activity when the monkey performed eye movements spontaneously outside learned behavioral tasks. However, the same neurons did change their spike activity when the monkey made a saccade in a purposeful way in a learned task; the change was always a decrease in discharge rate. In most cases the decrease in spike activity preceded the onset of a saccade and thereby could facilitate the initiation of a saccade.

The idea that the basal ganglia might be related to eye movement came from the discovery that the SNr has a fiber connection to the superior colliculus (*9*). In accordance with the anatomical data, neurons were found in the SNr that were activated antidromically from the superior colliculus (*7*). Such colliculus-projecting neurons were almost in variably related to saccades. We then compared the activities of the thus identified neuron pair and a striking feature became evident. While the SNr neuron was tonically active, the superior colliculus neuron was nearly silent. Before the saccade, the SNr neuron ceased discharging while the colliculus neuron showed a burst of spike activity. This result strongly suggested that the nigrocollicular connection is inhibitory, which concurred with other studies suggesting that the nigro-collicular connection is GABAergic (*16*). Because of the tonic inhibition, the superior colliculus neurons are disabled so that no saccade is elicited. Once the SNr neurons stop discharging and the tonic inhibition is removed, the superior colliculus neurons prepare to be excited and therefore are likely to produce a saccade.

The next question was how the SNr neurons stop discharging. The substantia nigra is known to receive massive fiber connections from other parts of the basal ganglia. The caudate nucleus is one such area (*1*). Unlike the SNr, the caudate is an extremely quiet area, and among the quiet neurons there, Hikosaka and Sakamoto (*2*) found saccade-related cells. They were clustered in the central region of the caudate which was elongated rostrocaudally. In order to test whether the saccadic signals in the caudate are sent to the SNr, we recorded single cell activity from the SNr and stimulated the caudate. Single pulse stimuli delivered in the saccade-related region, not outside of it, induced a clear inhibition in some neurons in the SNr. Most of the inhibited nigra neurons were related to saccades: they showed a decrease in spike activity before a saccade. Caudate neurons recorded close to the stimulating electrode were also saccade-related: they fired before a similar saccade. This experiment supports the hypothesis that the saccade-related decrease in nigra cell activity is caused by a phasic inhibition originating from the caudate nucleus.

From these experiments emerges a simple scheme. The caudate nucleus and the substantia nigra are both included in the basal ganglia. They constitute two serial inhibitions: caudate-nigral and nigro-collicular. The nigro-collicular inhibition is tonically active whereas the caudate-nigral inhibition becomes active only phasically. The tonic component acts to suppress the output. The second, phasic component opens the inhibitory gate, producing an output. In short, *disinhibition* is the way in which the basal ganglia act on the superior colliculus.

As I indicated before, the basal ganglia neurons were related only to those saccades that were made in behavioral paradigms. We trained our monkey to fixate on a small spot of light on the screen and to follow the movement of the spot by making eye movements. Two tasks were found to be quite useful; the saccade task was used to induce visually guided saccades, while the delayed saccade task was employed to induce memory-guided saccades. A number of caudate neurons were related to the saccade guided by the memory of a contralateral visual target. In the delayed saccade task, such a neuron started discharging near the end of the fixation period, and the discharge peaked with a saccade to the remembered position of the target. However, the neuron showed no discharge when saccades were made to the same target which was then actually present. The difference was surprising since the saccades in these two situations were nearly identical.

II. RELATION OF BASAL GANGLIA TO OTHER STRUCTURES

The basal ganglia interact with other brain areas in a number of ways; this is where this system reveals its unique role. The superior colliculus is the site where many different types of information converge (*17*): those from the retina and the cerebral cortex, including the visual cortex, parietal association cortex, and frontal eye field.

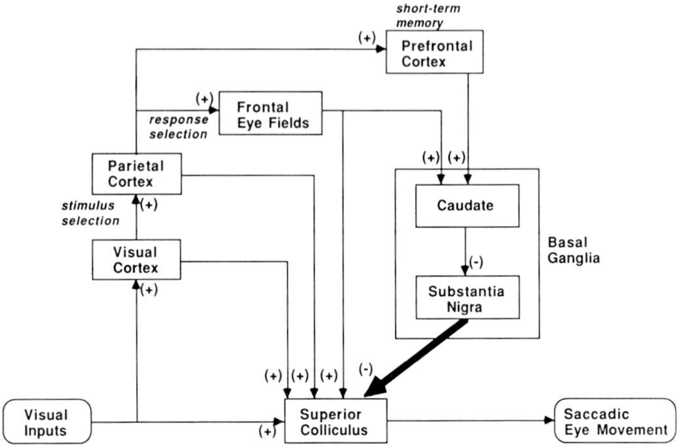

Fig. 1. Role of basal ganglia in initiation of saccadic eye movement. The basal ganglia system exerts its effect through disinhibition, while other structures have excitatory connections (+) to the superior colliculus. The substantia nigra normally exerts strong, tonic inhibition (−) on the superior colliculus, as indicated by a thickened arrow. Spontaneous activity in other connections is considered to be lower, as indicated by thin arrows.

The unique feature of the basal ganglia input is its suppressive nature (Fig. 1). Most of the other areas send the superior colliculus excitatory signals. Without the basal ganglia-induced inhibition, animals are forced to move eyes and other body parts incessantly. This was actually shown in our experiments in which the GABAergic nigro-collicular transmission was blocked (*8*). From such a chaotic urge to move emerges the necessity and importance of the basal ganglia suppressive mechanism.

Another important aspect is that the basal ganglia are primarily dominated by memory-dependent information, as shown for the caudate saccadic discharge, whereas the cerebral cortex is dominated by sensory information. The internal, memory-dependent information exerts its effect as a disinhibition through the basal ganglia, whereas the external, sensory-dependent information exerts its effect as an excitation directly from the cerebral cortex. They can be cooperative or competitive: cooperative if due to an excitation and a disinhibition, competitive if the basal ganglia-induced inhibition remains high or becomes even higher; the internal information would prevent sensory information from triggering movement.

The memory-oriented nature of the basal ganglia is also suggested by other types of cell activity. In addition to the saccade, we found visual, auditory, cognitive, and reward-related activities (*3*). Except for the auditory cells, these types were found close together with slight deviations. The same cells could show two, three or more types of activity, suggesting a clustering of cells that are functionally coupled. Even these sensory responses were often dependent on behavioral context; they appeared only in a particular situation of our saccade tasks. Most frequent among the activities classified as cognitive were those related to the expectation of task-related events. A considerable portion of caudate neurons exhibited activity before an external event, as if they knew what would happen next. With such predictive information, the basal ganglia might allow for the next movement awaiting triggering.

III. ROLE OF THE BASAL GANGLIA IN MOTOR PROGRAMMING

The question arises as to whether these anticipatory activities are used only in the preparation or initiation of movement. I have characterized the basal ganglia as a serial disinhibitory mechanism through which information is passed from the cerebral cortex to lower motor centers. However, if we look at the fiber connections of the basal ganglia, a different and more complex scheme emerges (Fig. 2). In addition to the superior colliculus, the substantia nigra projects to parts of the thalamus. These thalamic nuclei are mutually connected with the cerebral cortex (*12*). The cerebral cortex, especially the non-specific association cortex, also projects to the caudate (*11, 14*). These connections would complete the neural circuits involving the basal ganglia. Although admittedly oversimplified, this scheme gives us many hints as to how the basal ganglia might work.

The first hint derived from this scheme is that the basal ganglia has access to the neural events in the cerebral cortex. The basal

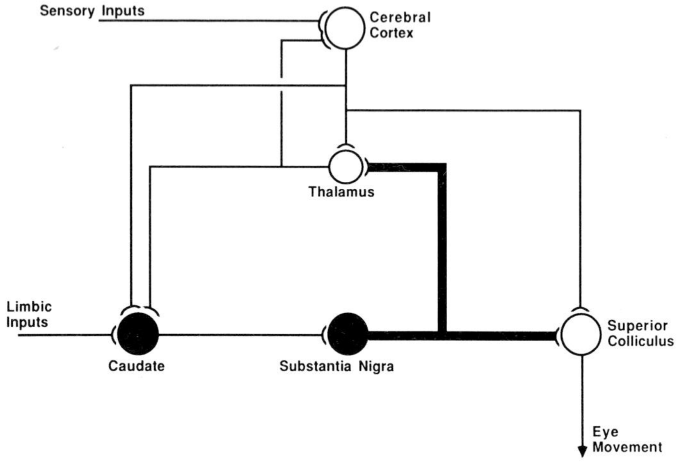

Fig. 2. Neural network loops composed of the cerebral cortex, thalamus, and the basal ganglia. The loops include two serial inhibitions, caudate-nigral and nigro-thalamic, as indicated by filled circles. The background level of nigro-thalamic and nigro-collicular inhibition is high, as indicated by thickened lines. How these networks might behave during learned motor behavior is discussed in the text.

ganglia activity may not simply be the result of cortical activities: it could itself exert an influence on the cerebral cortex. Here, I assume that the mutual connections between the thalamus and the cerebral cortex are excitatory. Also, I assume that there are excitatory mutual connections within the cerebral cortex.

The basal ganglia normally suppress the activity of thalamo-cortical circuits, but selectively release some of them. With a transient removal of inhibition, the thalamo-cortical activity may be set off so that it can be used for movement preparation or event anticipation. If we incorporate the pathway returning to the basal ganglia, yet another mode of basal ganglia operation can be pondered. This is a loop including two inhibitions which could act as a flip-flop circuit. In the resting state, the thalamo-cortical activity would be suppressed, and hence the caudate would receive no excitation; therefore, the substantia nigra activity would remain high and continue to suppress the thalamo-cortical activity. If somehow the caudate were excited, the substantia nigra output would be suppressed and the thalamo-cortical activity would be released from the inhibition. This state would be stable because the substantia nigra would be kept inhibited by the caudate. This mechanism would ensure that a selected cortical activity was maintained, perhaps until the next trigger signal was sent. Such a mechanism might be suggested by basal ganglia cell activity which is maintained until a task-specific event occurs. Different cells become active in sequence, punctuated by task-related events. If we delayed the appearance of the target, the cell activity would be prolonged accordingly.

Complex movements must be organized temporally as well as spatially. But is it really temporal organization that we need? We can see the sequence of neural activity, but the sequence may be independent of actual time. At the global level of learned behavior, a motor program or motor plan must be less dependent on time and more dependent on external events. Unlike reflexes, however, external events are always predicted; the brain does not respond but anticipates and confirms the ongoing behavioral contexts.

Here, the basal ganglia might come into play. The sequence of the motor program may exist in the cerebral cortex as a chain of excitatory connections. Such a neural chain alone would not work properly because its behavior would be heavily dependent on time. The key to overcoming such a difficulty might be found in the interaction with the basal ganglia. Suppose a unit in the cerebral cortex is active. The activity would be maintained through the cortico-basal ganglia loop, as I discussed earlier. The cortical activity is ready to be transmitted to the next unit. This would be prevented, however, by strong surrounding inhibition in the basal ganglia, which is known to be extensive in the striatum and substantia nigra (*10*). This state is therefore stable and less dependent on time.

If an expected event occurred, its signal would normally be fed into the next cortical unit, because this has already been learned. The brain just confirms the ongoing sequence. This would be good enough to transfer the active state to the next unit. Then the previously active unit as well as the next units would be suppressed by the surrounding inhibition in the basal ganglia. This process would continue, ensuring well-organized behavior.

SUMMARY

The basal ganglia contribute to the initiation of movements by disinhibition of target structures. The superior colliculus, as a saccade generator, is inhibited tonically by GABAergic connections from the substantia nigra pars reticulata. Phasic activity of caudate neurons, again through their GABAergic connections, suppresses the tonic nigral activity and thus leads to a disinhibition of superior colliculus cells. This disinhibition, in conjunction with other excitatory inputs, would produce burst activity, leading to a contralateral saccade. Inhibition is a unique feature of the basal ganglia. Another important aspect is that the basal ganglia are relatively dominated by memory-dependent information; external, sensory-dependent information has its effect as an excitation delivered directly from the cerebral cortex. In addition to the superior colliculus, the substantia nigra projects to parts of the thalamus which are mutually connected with the cerebral cortex. The basal ganglia would normally suppress the activity of thalamo-cortical circuits, but selectively release some of them. With a transient removal of inhibition, the thalamo-cortical activity may be set off so that it can be used for movement preparation or event anticipation. The connection is, in fact, closed since the cerebral cortex or the thalamus projects back to the caudate. These neural circuit loops are composed of two serial inhibitions in the basal ganglia and therefore might act to maintain the ongoing cortical activity. This would ensure stable execution of motor programming.

REFERENCES

1 Carpenter, M.B. (1981). In *Handbook of Physiology, The Nervous System*, vol. II, ed. Brooks, V.B., pp. 947–995. Bethesda, MD: American Physiological Society.
2 Hikosaka, O. and Sakamoto, M. (1986a). *Exp. Brain Res.* **63**, 659–662.
3 Hikosaka, O. and Sakamoto, M. (1986b). *Brain Dev.* **8**, 454–462.
4 Hikosaka, O. and Wurtz, R.H. (1983a). *J. Neurophysiol.* **49**, 1230–1253.
5 Hikosaka, O. and Wurtz, R.H. (1983b). *J. Neurophysiol.* **49**, 1254–1267.
6 Hikosaka, O. and Wurtz, R.H. (1983c). *J. Neurophysiol.* **49**, 1268–1284.
7 Hikosaka, O. and Wurtz, R.H. (1983d). *J. Neurophysiol.* **49**, 1285–1301.
8 Hikosaka, O. and Wurtz, R.H. (1985). *J. Neurophysiol.* **53**, 292–308.
9 Jayaraman, A., Batton, R.R., and Carpenter, M.B. (1977). *Brain Res.* **135**, 147–152.
10 Kitai, S.T. (1981). In *Handbook of Physiology, The Nervous System*, vol. II, ed. Brooks, V.B., pp. 997–1015. Bethesda, MD: American Physiological Society.
11 Percheron, G., Yelnik, J., and François, C. (1984). *J. Comp. Neurol.* **227**, 214–227.
12 Schell, G.R. and Strick, P.L. (1984). *J. Neurosci.* **4**, 539–560.
13 Scudder, C.A. (1988). *J. Neurophysiol.* **59**, 1455–1475.
14 Selemon, L.D. and Goldman-Rakic, P.S. (1985). *J. Neurosci.* **5**, 776–794.
15 Sparks, D.L. (1986). *Physiol. Rev.* **66**, 118–171.
16 Vincent, S.R., Hattori, T., and McGeer, E.G. (1978). *Brain Res.* **151**, 159–164.
17 Wurtz, R.H. and Albano, J.E. (1980). *Annu. Rev. Neurosci.* **3**, 189–226.

10

ACTIVITY OF THALAMIC NEURONS CONVEYING THE BASAL GANGLIA OUTPUT TO THE MOTOR CORTEX

KOHNOSUKE JINNAI,*[1] ATSUSHI NAMBU,*[2] AND SHIN-ICHI YOSHIDA*[2]

Department of Physiology, Shiga University of Medical Sciences, Ohtsu, Shiga 520-21,[1] Japan and Department of Physiology, Institute for Brain Research, Faculty of Medicine, Kyoto University, Kyoto 606,*[2] Japan*

Both the cerebellum and the basal ganglia send their output through the thalamus to the areas of the cerebral cortex which are related with the motor control function. It is widely accepted that the output from the cerebello-thalamic system exerts notable and direct influence on the movement control by the motor cortex. The influence of the pallido-thalamic system, however, is not as well understood as that of the cerebello-thalamic system. Recent electrophysiological studies in the behaving monkey revealed that many neurons in the globus pallidus change their discharge rate in synchrony with the movement of the limb and face muscles (*1*, *3*). If the movement-related activity of the pallidal neurons is relayed to the motor cortex through the thalamus, it is highly probable that the pallidal neurons exert a relatively direct influence on the activity of the muscles in the limb and face. However, the projection of the pallido-thalamic system directly to the motor cortex has not yet been unequivocally demonstrated. Recent anatomical studies reported that the internal segment of the globus pallidus (GPi) projects to the nucleus ventralis anterior pars parvocellularis (VApc) and nucleus ventralis lateralis pars oralis (VLo) in monkey thalamus (*5*). These thalamic nuclei are reported to project to the supplementary motor area (SMA) and the premotor area (*8*), but their projection to the motor cortex still appears to be controversial.

Using nonanesthetized monkeys as subjects, we recorded the activity of thalamic neurons which receive input from the GPi (GP-thalamic neurons). GP-thalamic neurons were found to project, not only to the premotor and SMA areas, but also to the motor cortex. GP-thalamic neurons projecting to the forelimb area of the motor cortex showed a movement-related discharge pattern similar to the discharge pattern of thalamic neurons receiving input from the cerebellar nuclei (CN-thalamic neurons). These findings suggest that the output through the pallidothalamic system to the motor cortex plays an important and direct role in the control of limb movement.

I. PROJECTION OF GP-THALAMIC NEURONS TO THE MOTOR CORTEX

We employed the following procedures to determine the area of the cerebral cortex to which each thalamic neuron is projected, and to identify the input to the neuron from the GPi or cerebellar nuclei (CN). Concentric electrodes were permanently implanted in the

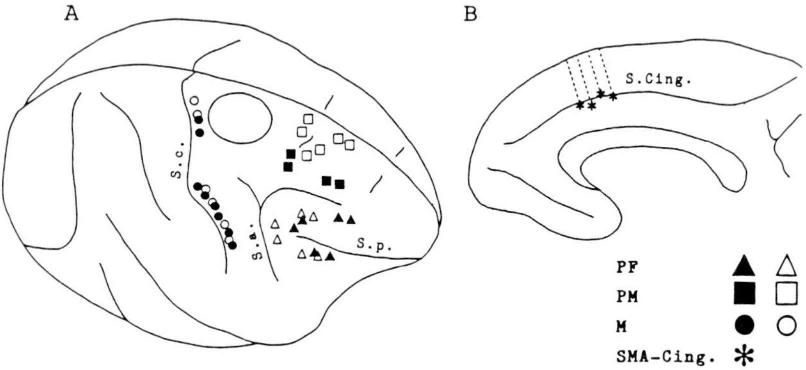

Fig. 1. Illustrations showing the location of the bipolar stimulating electrodes in the cerebral cortex. Dorsolateral (A) and mesial (B) views of the right cerebral hemisphere. Black and white symbols represent the electrodes in the two different monkeys. S.c.: central sulcus, S.p.: principal sulcus, S.a.: arcuate sulcus, S.Cing.: cingulate sulcus. The oval shape on the premotor area indicates the placement of the recording chamber.

external (GPe) and internal (GPi) segments of the GP, and the CN of two Japanese monkeys. Bipolar stimulating electrodes were also implanted into various areas of the cerebral cortex, such as the motor (area 4), premotor and prefrontal areas. In one monkey, additional bipolar electrodes were implanted into the dorsal and ventral banks of the cingulate sulcus to stimulate both the SMA and the cingulate area (SMA-cingulate area) (see Fig. 1). A few weeks after the implantation, activities of the thalamic neurons were recorded with a glass-coated elgiloy microelectrode, which was introduced vertically through the recording chamber.

Input from the GPi to a thalamic neuron was examined by suppression of spontaneous discharges due to stimulation of the GPi using an intensity less than 0.5 mA (0.3 msec duration). Figure 2C shows an example of the suppression induced by the GPi stimulation. Activities of 92 of the 162 thalamocortical neurons examined were suppressed by GPi stimulation. The latency of the suppression was less than 2.5 msec in most (86%) of the 92 neurons. The possibility that the suppression was produced by the current spread of the GPi stimulation to the surrounding structures was excluded, because the stimulation through the electrode located in the GPe (GP3 in Fig. 2F), or in the medial part of the GPi close to the internal capsule (GP1 in G) was less effective than the stimulation through the electrode in the center of the GPi(GP2). Input from the CN to a thalamic neuron was examined by orthodromic discharges after stimulation of the CN.

The area in the cerebral cortex to which a thalamic neuron projected was determined by an antidromic response to stimulation of the cerebral cortex with a current pulse of 0.5mA, 0.3 msec duration. Almost all (309/313) of the thalamocortical neurons were activated antidromically with only one pair of bipolar electrodes, but these neurons were not activated by other electrodes about 3 mm apart. This indicated that the stimulus did not effectively spread more than 1.5 mm. Figure 2 shows a GP-thalamic neuron which was activated antidromically by stimulation of the forelimb area in the motor cortex. The threshold of the antidromic response of this neuron elicited by stimulating the electrode in the rostral bank of the central sulcus (Fig. 2, E) was less than 0.2mA. This finding indicates that the GP-thalamic neuron projects to the motor cortex.

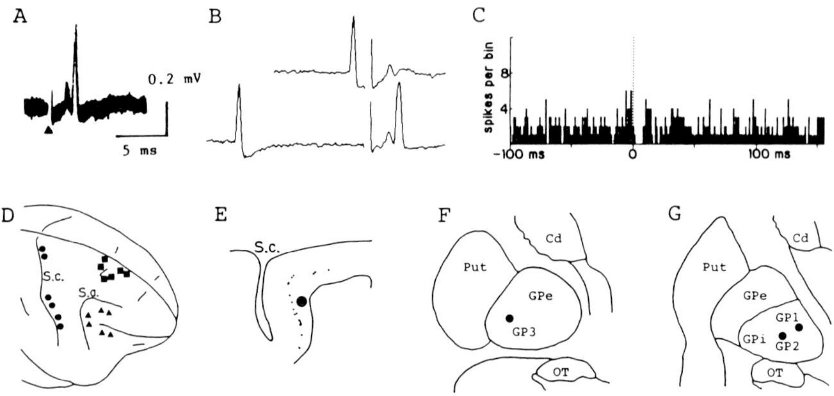

Fig. 2. A: antidromic response induced by stimulation of the forelimb area of the motor cortex. B: collision of the antidromic response of the above-described neuron with the preceding spontaneous discharges (average of 10 sweeps triggered by spontaneous discharges). C: post-stimulus time histogram (PSTH) showing suppression of spontaneous discharges of the above neuron after GPi stimulation at time 0 (55 sweeps, bin width 1 msec). D: surface view of the cerebral hemisphere showing the location of the stimulating electrodes. E: location of tip of the stimulating electrode in the forelimb area of the motor cortex in a parasagittal section (right side, rostral). F and G: location of stimulating electrodes in the external (F) and internal (G) segments of GP shown in frontal sections.

TABLE I
Number of Thalamic Neurons Which Receive Input from the GPi, CN, or Both (GPi+CN), and Project to Different Cortical Areas

		(Cortical projection area)				
		PF	PM	SMA-Cing.	M	Total
(input)	GPi	4	21	20	44	89
	GPi+CN				3	3
	CN		5	2	63	70

PF: prefrontal area, PM: premotor area, SMA-Cing.: SMA-cingulate area, M: motor cortex (area 4).

Table I shows the number of GP- and CN-thalamic neurons projecting to different areas of the cerebral cortex. Activities of 89 thalamic neurons of the 162 neurons examined were suppressed by the GPi stimulation, but were not activated by the CN stimulation. Of the 89 neurons, 44 projected to the motor cortex. The number of GP-thalamic neurons projecting to the motor cortex was larger than expected.

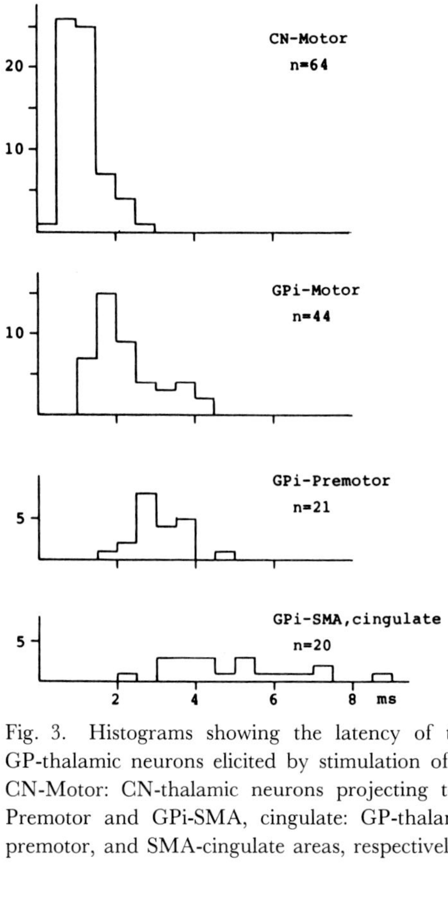

Fig. 3. Histograms showing the latency of the antidromic response of CN- and GP-thalamic neurons elicited by stimulation of different areas of the cerebral cortex. CN-Motor: CN-thalamic neurons projecting to the motor cortex. GPi-Motor, GPi-Premotor and GPi-SMA, cingulate: GP-thalamic neurons projecting to the motor, premotor, and SMA-cingulate areas, respectively.

The number of thalamic neurons which received inputs from both the CN and GPi was very small (3/162). This coincides well with the result of a previous electrophysiological study in the squirrel monkey (*10*).

GP-thalamic neurons projecting to the motor cortex were located mainly in the VLo, and those projecting to the premotor and SMA-cingulate areas were frequently found in the VApc. CN-thalamic neurons projecting to the motor cortex were located mainly in the nucleus ventralis posterior lateralis pars oralis (VPLo) and nuclues ventralis pars caudalis (VLc) (see ref. *6*). The location of the GP-thalamic neurons also corresponds well to the distribution of the terminals of the pallidothalamic projection fibers (*5*). These findings appear to indicate that the suppression of discharges induced by GPi stimulation is due to activation of the pallidothalamic neurons.

Figure 3 shows the latencies of the antidromic responses of the different neuronal groups. The antidromic latency of the GP-thalamic neurons projecting to the motor cortex (mean: 2.2 ± 0.79 msec) is significantly longer than that of the CN-thalamic neurons projecting to the same area (1.1 ± 0.44 msec), yet it is shorter than that of the GP-thalamic neurons proejcting to the premotor area (3.0 ± 1.6 msec). The difference in the antidromic latency and location between GP-thalamic neurons projecting to the motor cortex and those projecting to the premotor area supports the view that the antidromic response elicited by stimulation of the motor cortex is not due to current spread to the neighboring premotor area.

II. DISCHARGE PATTERN OF GP-THALAMIC NEURONS

Changes in the discharge rate of GP-thalamic neurons and CN-thalamic neurons during the performance of a reaction time task were compared. Two monkeys were trained to lift a lever using dorsiflexion of their wrist joint, within 500 msec duration of light stimulus. Figure 4 shows examples of GP-thalamic (A) and CN-thalamic (B) neurons. Both neurons were antidromically activated by stimulation of the forelimb area of the motor cortex, as shown in A, a and B, a. The GP-thalamic neuron in A increased its discharge rate 110 msec prior to the onset of lever-lifting movement (c). The CN-thalamic neuron in B showed a similar discharge pattern (c). Ten out of 18 GP-thalamic neurons projecting to the forelimb area of the motor cortex increased (9/10) or decreased (1/10) their discharge rate synchronously with the lever-lifting movement. These neurons showed changes in the discharge rate, not only in the course of the reaction time task, but also when the lever-lifting movement was initiated spontaneously (self-initiated movement). These changes in the discharge rate were regarded as a movement-related discharge pattern. Of the 34 CN-thalamic neurons projecting to the forelimb area of the motor cortex, the discharge rate of 33 neurons changed in a similar manner. The incidence of GP-thalamic neurons with the

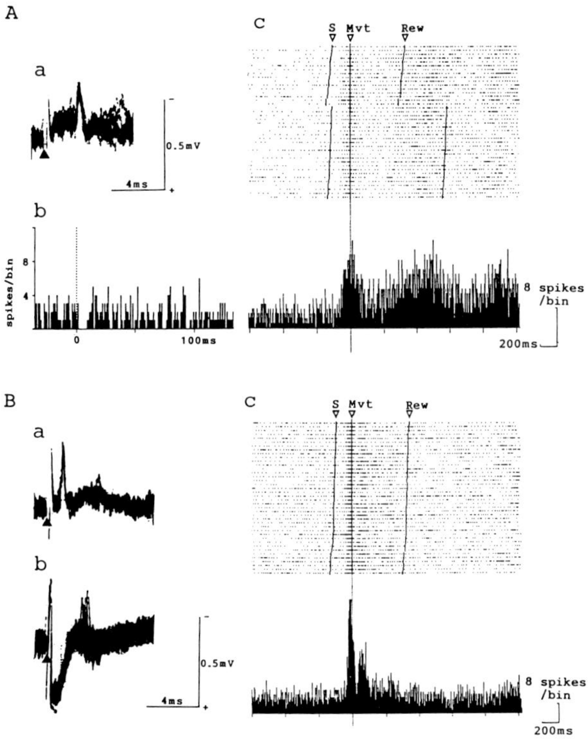

Fig. 4. Two examples (A and B) of thalamic neurons with input from GPi or CN. A, a: antidromic response elicited by stimulation of the forelimb area of the motor cortex. b: PSTH showing suppression of discharges of the above neuron after GPi-stimulation. c: raster display and frequency histogram of unitary discharges of the above neuron during the performance of the reaction time task. S, light stimuli, Mvt, onset of movement, Rew, reward. Trials were arranged in the order of reaction times. Timing of the reward was varied in order to examine the relation between the later increase in the discharge rate and the reward. B, a: antidromic response to stimulation of the forelimb area of the motor cortex. b: orthodromic response of the same neuron to CN-stimulation. c: raster display and histogram of discharge of the same neuron.

movement-related discharge pattern seemed lower than that in CN-thalamic neurons.

The time between the onset of change in the discharge rate of thalamic neurons and the onset of movement in one monkey is plotted in Fig. 5, along with the EMG activities of several muscles. EMG activity of the m. brachioradialis was initiated earlier than any of the other muscles recorded, such as m. biceps brachii, m. triceps

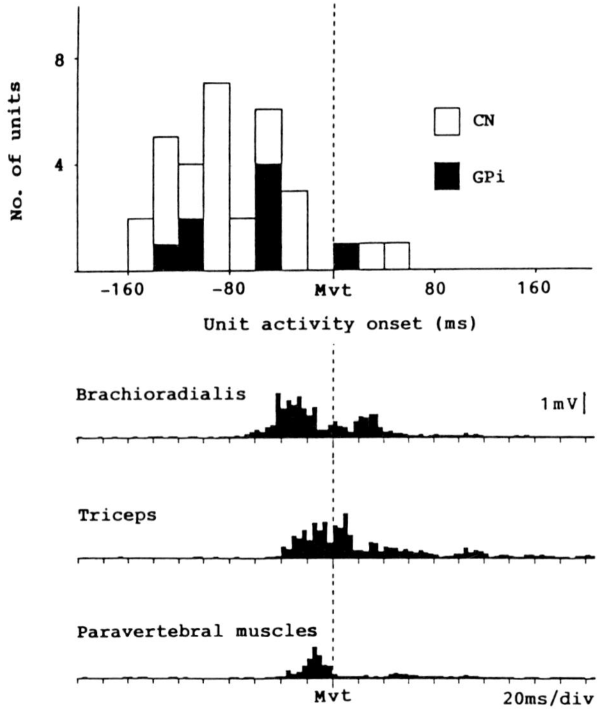

Fig. 5. Histogram of the onset time of activity change of thalamic neurons before and after the onset of the lever-lifting movement during the course of the reaction time task. Black and white squares represent GP- and CN-thalamic neurons, respectively. All thalamic neurons were recorded from one monkey, and were found to project to the forelimb area of the motor cortex. Lower traces show the changes in amplitude of the rectified EMG during the performance of the same task (average of 10 trials).

brachii, muscles in the shoulder and back, and the wrist flexor muscles. This histogram shows that the onset time of activity change in the two types of thalamic neurons did not differ significantly.

The discharge rates of some of the GP-thalamic neurons were changed, more than 30 msec prior to the onset of the EMG activity. Fetz and Cheney, using the spike-triggered averaging technique, observed facilitation of the EMG activity following the spike discharges of single neurons in the motor cortex (post-spike facilitation), and the onset latencies of the post-spike facilitation for most of the corticomotoneuronal cells were reported to be less than 20 msec (mean latency: 6.7 msec) (*2*). Therefore, the value of 30 msec seems long enough for these GP-thalamic neurons to contribute to the initiation of the movement.

III. CHARACTERISTICS OF GP-THALAMIC NEURONS PROJECTING TO AREAS OTHER THAN THE MOTOR CORTEX

GP-thalamic neurons projecting to the premotor and SMA-cingulate areas were located in the more rostral part of the thalamus (VApc), and their axons revealed slower conduction velocities than CN- and GP-thalamic neurons projecting to the motor cortex. Only a few of these thalamic neurons showed the movement-related discharge pattern. These results suggest that the functional role of the pallidothalamic system projecting to the premotor and SMA-cingulate areas is quite different from that of the system projecting to the motor cortex. Thalamic neurons of the cat which receive inhibitory input from the entopeduncular nucleus (ENT-thalamic neurons) showed characteristics similar to the GP-thalamic neurons projecting to the premotor and SMA-cingulate areas in the monkey. A previous study by the present authors (*4*) showed that ENT-thalamic neurons project mainly to the medial part of the anterior sigmoid cortex, which corresponds to area 6, and that their axons have slow conduction velocity (mean antidromic latency: 6.1 ± 3.9 msec). Almost all (13/14) of the ENT-thalamic neurons were found to project to layer I of the anterior sigmoid cortex; they were antidromically activated by weak microstimulation (less than 35 μA) in layer I. It would be reasonable to assume that the axons of the GP-thalamic neurons projecting to the premotor and SMA-cingulate areas of the monkey also terminate in layer I. If they projected to layer I, they would generate excitatory postsynaptic potentials (EPSPs) on the distal part of the apical dendrites of the cortical pyramidal neurons. Such EPSPs may be less effective in producing a rapid increase in the discharge rate, but suitable for producing a gradual and sustained increase in the discharge rate of the cortical pyramidal neurons. It was reported that some neurons in the premotor area (*9*) and the SMA (*7*) showed a sustained increase in the discharge rate during the delay period between the instruction signal and movement triggering signal. It is probable that the GP-thalamic neurons projecting to the premotor area and SMA contribute to the generation of such sustained activities of the cortical neurons in these areas.

SUMMARY

Unitary activities of thalamic neurons were studied in nonanesthetized monkeys. Stimulating electrodes were permanently implanted in various areas of the cerebral cortex, basal ganglia, and cerebellum of monkeys. Thalamic neurons with input from the globus pallidus (GP-thalamic neurons) and those with input from the cerebellar nuclei (CN-thalamic neurons) were identified by their inhibitory and excitatory responses to stimulation of the internal segment of the GP and the CN, respectively. Cortical projection areas of these thalamic neurons were determined by an antidromic response of the respective neurons to localized stimulation of the cerebral cortex. GP-thalamic neurons were found to project, not only to the premotor and supplementary motor areas, but also to the motor cortex (area 4). About half (10/18) of the GP-thalamic neurons projecting to the forelimb area of the motor cortex changed their discharge rate synchronously with the movement, in the same manner as most (33/34) of the CN-thalamic neurons projecting to the same area. Few of the GP-thalamic projecting to the premotor, supplementary motor or cingulate area revealed this type of movement-related discharge pattern, and their axons exhibited a slow conduction velocity. These findings suggest that the output from the pallidothalamic system to the motor cortex plays, at least in part, a direct role in the control of movement. The pallido-thalamic system projecting to the premotor and supplementary motor areas, however, might contribute to motor control in an indirect way.

REFERENCES

1 DeLong, M.R., Crutcher, M.D., and Georgopoulos, A.P. (1985). *J. Neurophysiol.* **53**, 530–543.
2 Fetz, E.E. and Cheney, P.D. (1980). *J. Neurophysiol.* **44**, 751–772.
3 Georgopoulos, A.P., DeLong, M.R., and Crutcher, M.D. (1983). *J. Neurosci.* **3**, 1586–1598.

4 Jinnai, K. Nambu, A., and Yoshida, S. (1987). *Exp. Brain Res.* **69**, 67-76.
5 Kim. R., Nakano, K., Jayaraman, A., and Carpenter, M.B. (1976). *J. Comp. Neurol.* **169**, 263-290.
6 Nambu, A., Yoshida, S., and Jinnai, K. (1988). *Exp. Brain Res.* **71**, 656-662.
7 Romo, R. and Schultz, W. (1984). *Exp. Brain Res.* **67**, 656-662.
8 Schell, G.R. and Strick, P.L. (1984). *J. Neurosci.* **4**, 539-560.
9 Weinrich, M., Wise, S.P., and Mauritz, K.H. (1984). *Brain* **107**, 385-414.
10 Yamamoto, T., Hassler, R., Huber, C., Wagner, A., and Sasaki, K. (1983). *Exp. Brain Res.* **51**, 77-87.

PROGRAMMING IN THE VISUAL SYSTEM

11

NEURAL COMMANDS FOR THE CONTROL OF SACCADIC EYE MOVEMENTS: REQUIRED TRANSFORMATIONS OF SIGNALS OBSERVED IN THE SUPERIOR COLLICULUS

DAVID L. SPARKS

Neurobiology Research Center, Department of Physiology and Biophysics, University of Alabama at Birmingham, Birmingham, Alabama 35294, U.S.A.

Because of their extremely high velocity and remarkable precision, neurophysiologists have a long-standing interest in the neural control of saccadic eye movements. Quantitative descriptions of the discharge patterns of the motoneurons innervating the extraocular muscles have been obtained from chronic unit recording experiments. Neural circuits involving cells in the pons, medulla and midbrain have been identified that form the command signals observed at the motoneuron level. At a higher level, an accumulating body of evidence (*38*) suggests that command signals for the initiation of saccadic eye movements are generated in the superior colliculus (SC).

The purpose of this paper is to: a) describe the saccadic command signals observed in the deep layers of the SC; b) describe current models of the brainstem circuits forming the signals recorded from motoneurons; and c) speculate on the loci and mechanisms of the transformations of collicular signals required to interface with these brainstem circuits.

I. SIGNALS OBSERVED IN THE SUPERIOR COLLICULUS

Saccade-related burst neurons (SRBNs) in the deep layers of the SC generate a discrete, high-frequency burst of spike activity beginning 18–20 msec before saccade onset (*40*). The discharge of SRBNs is not related to moving the eye to a particular position in the orbit but to certain changes in eye position (*34, 40, 44*). Each SRBN has a movement field, *i.e.*, each cell discharges before a range of saccades that have particular directions and amplitudes (*40, 44*). The SRBNs are arranged topographically according to the location of their movement fields and, thereby, form a map of saccadic motor error, *i.e.*, a map of the distance and direction of the saccade required to look to a target.

Since each SRBN fires before a broad range of saccades, a large population of collicular neurons discharges before each saccade (*24, 40*). A spatial and temporal distribution of activity is observed in this active population. Neurons in the center of the population fire earlier and more vigorously; cells on the fringe of the active population fire weakly and their activity may follow, rather than precede, saccade onset (*39*). But the discharge of a single collicular neuron is ambiguous with respect to saccade direction or amplitude. Each SRBN generates identical discharges before many saccades with different directions and amplitudes (*39*). Thus, the discharge of a single collicular neuron cannot specify the direction and amplitude of an impending saccade. Instead, information about the direction and amplitude of a saccade is encoded anatomically by the location of the active neurons within the motor map contained in the SC. Recent evidence suggests that the level of activity within the active population may be a determinant of saccadic velocity (*2, 32*).

To summarize, the activity of neurons in the SC specifies the desired change in eye position, not a movement to a particular position in the orbit. Saccade direction and amplitude are encoded anatomically. It is the location of active neurons within the topographical map of movement fields, not their frequency of firing, that specifies the trajectory of a saccade. Saccadic velocity may be encoded by the frequency of firing of the population of active neurons.

II. FORMATION OF THE MOTONEURON SIGNAL

A high frequency burst of motoneuron activity precedes saccade onset by about 8 msec (*11*, *29*, *33*). For small saccades, the frequency of the motoneuron burst is related to saccadic velocity and amplitude. But for saccades larger than 10°, burst frequency saturates and becomes unrelated to saccadic amplitude. Because of this saturation, the major determinant of saccadic amplitude for large saccades is burst duration. The burst of activity is not a rectangular pulse, but decays with a short and a long time constant to the steady-state level of activity associated with the new position (*11*, *29*). Thus, the pattern of activity observed at the single motoneuron level is a pulse/slide/step waveform, a pattern of innervation required by Robinson's early model (*28*) of the oculomotor plant.

Most researchers assume that neural circuits located in the brainstem perform the computations required to form commands appropriate for each of the extraocular muscles (see ref. *12* for a recent review). Neurons located in the pontine and medullary reticular formation are thought to generate signals responsible for the horizontal component of saccadic eye movements (see below) while neurons in the rostral midbrain control the vertical components (*4*, *5*).

The local feedback scheme proposed by Robinson (*30*, *42*) was the earliest model of a brainstem circuit for generating the pulse/step innervation signal. The model only considers horizontal saccades and is based upon the properties of cells found in the pontine reticular formation (*16*, *21*): medium-lead burst neurons (MLBs); omnipause neurons (OPNs); and tonic neurons (TNs). MLBs generate a high-frequency burst before ipsilateral saccades. OPNs fire at a relatively constant rate during fixation and pause during saccades in all directions. It is assumed that OPNs exert a powerful inhibition upon MLB neurons since electrical stimulation in the vicinity of OPNs prevents the occurrence of saccadic eye movements. TNs discharge at a frequency proportional to horizontal eye position and are thought to provide the step component of motoneuron firing. It is assumed that the firing of TNs represents the output of a neural integrator that converts the saccadic pulse into a step signal.

According to the model, there are two inputs to this brainstem circuit: a signal of the desired position of the eye and a trigger signal. Saccades are initiated by the trigger signal that briefly inhibits the OPNs. This permits MLBs to discharge at a rate proportional to motor error (the difference between the desired position and an internal estimate of current eye position). The pulse of activity generated by MLBs is transmitted directly to motoneurons and to a neural integrator (NI). The NI converts the pulse into a step of activity that is sent to motoneurons and used as the estimate of current eye position. Once activated, this circuit drives the eye at a high velocity until the representation of current position matches the signal of desired position. At that point, the eye stops on target, and the OPNs are allowed to resume firing. The discharge of the OPNs inactivates the pulse/step generator until a new trigger signal arrives.

Modifications of Robinson's model have been proposed by several investigators (*1, 18, 36, 41*). In part, these modifications were attempts to design models consistent with the signals observed in the SC and frontal eye fields, structures known to be critical for saccade generation (*15, 35*). Neurons in these areas generate commands for *changes* in eye position or *desired displacement*, rather than commands to move the eye to a particular position in the orbit. Accordingly, a common characteristic of the alternative models is that MLBs are driven by a signal specifying the *desired change in eye position* rather than a signal of the desired absolute position of the eye in the orbit.

Thus, according to these models, only two input signals are required by each brainstem pulse/step generator circuit, a trigger signal and a signal of desired orbital position (Robinson) or desired displacement (modified models). Note, however, that most of the models do not generate oblique saccades (saccades having both horizontal and vertical components). Also, they assume that all saccades start with the eye in the center of the orbit. These points are discussed in more detail below.

III. REQUIRED TRANSFORMS

1. Trigger Signal

As noted above, models of the pulse/step generator require a trigger signal to briefly inhibit the OPN. The discharge of SRBNs found in the SC could serve as the trigger input to pulse/step generator circuits. The high-frequency burst of SRBNs is tightly linked to saccade onset and precedes saccade onset by an appropriate time, approximately 20 ms. Consistent with the features of the trigger signal, SRBNs signal saccade onset not saccade direction, amplitude, or duration. The axons of SRBNs probably comprise a major efferent pathway from SC to subsequent oculomotor premotor neurons, particularly the PPRF (*26*). Keller (*17*) reported that 10 of 10 SRBNs recorded in the SC were antidromically activated by stimulation of the region of the PPRF containing OPNs. Only 1 of 11 other collicular neurons with saccade-related discharges, but lacking the high-frequency burst, was antidromically activated by PPRF stimulation.

2. Signal of Desired Orbital Position or Desired Change in Position

Models of the pulse/step generator also require signals of the desired position of the eye in the orbit or a signal of the desired change in position. Note, however, that while the activity of most neurons in the SC is related to both horizontal and vertical components, separate pulse/step generators exist for the control of the horizontal and vertical components of a saccade. Thus, separate signals of horizontal motor error (ME) and vertical ME must be extracted from the anatomical map of vectorial ME found in the colliculus.

Recent experiments suggest that neurons in the central midbrain reticular formation (cMRF) could be involved in extracting information about the horizontal component of oblique saccades (*7*). Neurons in the intermediate and deeper layers of the SC project to the cMRF (*6*) and, in turn, neurons in the cMRF project to regions of the pontine reticular formation involved in the control of horizontal saccades (*9*). Cells in the cMRF burst before contralateral saccades having horizontal components and microstimulation in this area only

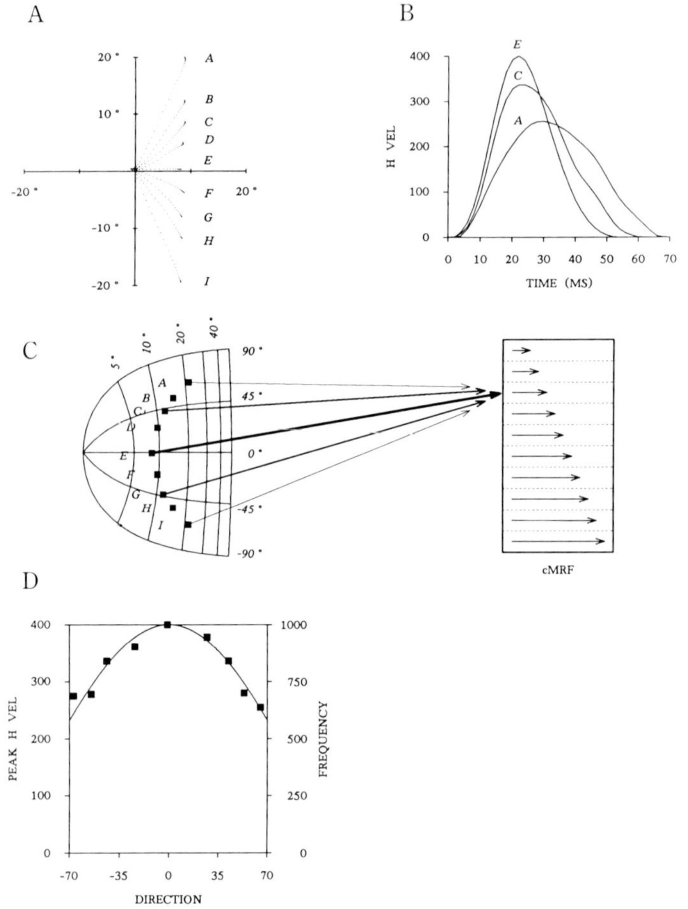

Fig. 1. A: trajectories of 9 saccades having the same horizontal amplitude. B: velocity profiles of the horizontal component of 3 of the saccades shown in A. Note that the horizontal component of saccade E (no vertical component) has the highest velocity and the shortest duration. The horizontal components of oblique saccades C and A have lower velocities and longer durations. C: on the left is a representation of the motor map found in the left SC. Iso-direction lines (0, 45, 90) and iso-amplitude lines (5, 10, 20, 40) are shown. The filled squares show the sites of maximal neuronal activity associated with each of the saccades illustrated in panel A. The rectangle on the right represents the cMRF. Top is dorsal; bottom is ventral. Stimulation dorsally produces small horizontal saccades (short arrows). Stimulation ventrally produces large horizontal saccades (longer arrows). Each neuron along an iso-ΔH line projects to neurons at the same depth in the cMRF, as illustrated by the arrows. The width of the lines represents the strength of the synaptic connections between neurons in the SC and neurons in the cMRF. D: the solid line represents the firing rate of a single neuron in the cMRF for saccades of different

produces horizontal saccades (*43*). The amplitude of the stimulation-induced horizontal movement depends upon the depth of the stimulating electrode. Small amplitude movements are evoked by stimulation dorsally and progressively larger movements are evoked as the electrode is moved ventrally (*8, 43*).

Based upon these findings, Sparks (*38*) proposed a method for extracting a signal of horizontal ME from the anatomically coded signals observed in the SC. Figure 1A displays the trajectory of 9 saccades having a 10° rightward horizontal component but differing in direction and total (vectorial) amplitude. Figure 1C (left) illustrates the locations of the neurons in the SC that discharge maximally before the 9 saccades shown in A. If the axons of all the collicular neurons residing along this iso-ΔH curve (same change in horizontal position) converged upon neurons at a specific depth in the cMRF (Fig. 1C, right), neurons at that depth would discharge before any saccade having a 10° horizontal component. According to this scheme, neurons residing at other depths in the cMRF would receive signals from collicular neurons residing along different iso-ΔH curves. Information about the vertical component of oblique saccades could be extracted in a similar fashion by tectorecipient neurons in another (unknown) nucleus. Cohen and Buttner-Ennever (*6*) observed differential retrograde labelling in rostral and caudal SC following injection of anatomical tracer material into dorsal and ventral cMRF, but their data cannot be used in support of this hypothesis since they did not look for the specific pattern of label suggested by Fig. 1.

In summary, specific patterns of anatomical connections between neurons in the SC and cMRF provide a mechanism for extracting information about the horizontal component of saccadic eye movements. Additional anatomical and electrophysiological experiments are needed as tests of this hypothesis.

---

directions, all of which have the same horizontal amplitude. The solid squares represent the peak velocity of the horizontal component of the saccades illustrated in A. Appropriate weighting of synaptic connections between SC and cMRF would yield neurons in the cMRF with firing rates proportional to the velocity of the horizontal component of oblique saccades.

3. Coordination of the Horizontal and Vertical Components of Oblique Saccades

The separate signals of horizontal and vertical ME must be coordinated in order to produce oblique saccades. Oblique saccades usually have relatively straight (rather than curved) trajectories (Fig. 1A) because the onsets of the horizontal and vertical pulses are synchronized and the durations of the horizontal and vertical displacements are approximately equal (*20*). When the amplitudes of the horizontal and vertical components of an oblique saccade are unequal, the duration of the smaller component is greater than the duration of a pure horizontal or vertical saccade of the same amplitude (Fig. 1B). The increased duration of the minor component of oblique saccades is neurally mediated; abducens neurons (*20*) and midbrain MLBs (*19*) display a decrease in average firing rate and an increase in burst duration under these conditions. This implies that signals controlling the velocity of the horizontal and vertical components of oblique saccades are based upon the amplitude of the total movement.

The hypothesis presented in Fig. 1 can be extended to suggest a mechanism by which component velocity could be scaled according to saccadic direction. Neurons encoding the velocity of the horizontal component of oblique saccades by their frequency of firing could be formed by allowing cMRF cells to receive excitatory synaptic inputs from all members of an iso-ΔH curve, but scaling the strength of the excitation by the location of collicular cell along the curve (Fig. 1C). For example, those members of the 5° iso-ΔH curve that are located rostrally and near the middle of the colliculus (cells associated with 5° horizontal movements having no vertical component) would provide greater excitatory drive than members located more caudally and medially or laterally (*i.e.*, cells associated with 5° horizontal movements and large vertical components). Appropriate scaling of synaptic strength according to the location of neurons in the SC would permit cMRF cells to fire at frequencies proportional to the velocity of the horizontal component of oblique saccades (Fig. 1D).

4. Compensation for the Origin and Endpoint of Saccades

The saccadic command observed in the SC needs to be supplemented by signals compensating for the orbital position of the origin and endpoint of a saccade. The total pulse of innervation provided by motoneuron pools must vary considerably for identical saccades with different starting positions (*31*). Saccades to visual targets compensate for the position of the eye in the orbit and the cerebellum is involved in the generation of signals to compensate for position-dependent viscous and elastic forces (*25, 27*). Apparently, these compensatory signals are not added when saccades are produced by collicular stimulation (*37*; Sparks, unpublished observations). For example, stimulation of a collicular site that produces a purely horizontal saccade 10° in amplitude when the eye is in the center of the orbit will produce a saccade with a small downward component if the eye is elevated and a small upward component if, prior to stimulation, the eye is rotated downward. Similarly, centrifugal stimulation-induced saccades are smaller than centripetal ones.

Although not studied exhaustively, neither the saccade-related discharge of collicular neurons (*40, 44*) nor the discharge of MLBs in the PPRF (*16, 42*) vary depending upon initial eye position. It is possible that a neural circuit involving neurons in the nucleus reticularis tegmenti pontis (NRTP) and cerebellar vermis are involved in the generation of a compensatory signal. The region of the NRTP containing cells with saccade-related activity receives extensive projections from the intermediate layers of the SC (*14*) and sends a majority, if not all, of its efferent projections to the cerebellum (*3, 13*). Cells in the NRTP with saccade-related activity have movement fields similar to those described for cells in the SC (*10*), but the vigor of the burst of NRTP cells differs depending upon the origin of the movement (*10*). Also, neurons in the cerebellar vermis display eye-position dependent variations in saccade-related bursts (*22, 23*).

SUMMARY

The saccadic command signals observed in the SC differ from those required by the motoneurons and a number of transformations are required. Figure 2 summarizes the speculations presented in this paper. Collicular signals are transmitted simultaneously *via* parallel pathways to several brainstem sites. The current working hypothesis

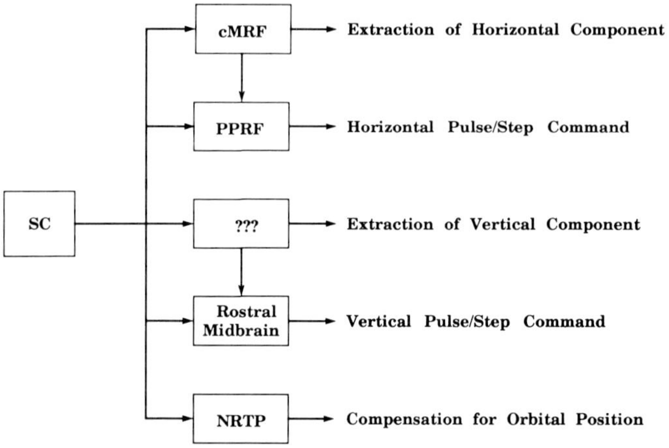

Fig. 2. A schematic diagram of the hypothesized location of neurons involved in transforming collicular signals.

in our laboratory is that the major tectorecipient areas outlined in Fig. 2 specialize in one or more of the following signal transformations: the generation of separate ME signals for the horizontal and vertical pulse/step generators; the formation of signals to control the velocity of the horizontal and vertical components of oblique saccades; and the development of signals to correct for position-dependent viscous and elastic forces of the eye.

Acknowledgments
The work cited from this laboratory was supported by grants from the National Institutes of Health (R01-EY01189, R01-EY05486, and P30-EY03039) and a grant from the Alfred P. Sloan Foundation.

REFERENCES

1 Becker, W. and Jurgens, R. (1979). *Vision Res.* **19**, 976–983.
2 Berthoz, A., Grantyn, A., and Droulez, J. (1986). *Neurosci. Lett.* **72**, 289–294.
3 Brodal, A. and Jansen, J. (1946). *J. Comp. Neurol.* **84**, 31–118.
4 Buttner, U., Buttner-Ennever, J.A. and Henn, V. (1977). *Brain Res.* **130**, 239–252.
5 Buttner-Ennever, J.A. and Buttner, U. (1978). *Brain Res.* **151**, 31–47.

6 Cohen, B. and Buttner-Ennever, J.A. (1984) *Exp. Brain Res.* **57**, 167–176.
7 Cohen, B., Matsuo, V., Raphan, T., Waitzman, D., and Fradin, J. (1982) In *Physiological and Pathological Aspects of Eye Movements*, ed. Roucoux, A. and Crommelinck, M., pp. 325–335. The Hague: Dr. W. Junk.
8 Cohen, B., Matsuo, V., Fradin, J., and Raphan, T. (1985). *Exp. Brain Res.* **57**, 605–616.
9 Cohen, B., Waitzman, D., Buttner-Ennever, J., and Matsuo, V. (1986). In *Progress in Brain Research*, vol. 64, ed. Freund, H.-J., Buttner, V., Cohen, B., and Noth, J., pp. 243–256. Amsterdam, New York: Elsevier.
10 Crandall, W.F. and Keller, E.L. (1985). *J. Neurophysiol.* **54**, 1326–1345.
11 Fuchs, A.F. and Luschei, E.S. (1970). *J. Neurophysiol.* **33**, 382–392.
12 Fuchs, A.F., Kaneko, C.R.S., and Scudder, C.A. (1985) *Annu. Rev. Neurosci.* **8**, 307–337.
13 Gerrits, N.M. and Voogd, J. (1986). *Exp. Brain Res.* **62**, 29–45.
14 Harting, J.K. (1977). *J. Comp. Neurol.* **173**, 583–612.
15 Hikosaka, O. and Wurtz, R.H. (1985). *J. Neurophysiol.* **53**, 266–291.
16 Keller, E.L. (1974). *J. Neurophysiol.* **37**, 316–332.
17 Keller, E.L. (1979). In *Progress in Brain Research. Reflex Control of Posture and Movement*, ed. Granit, R. and Pompeiano, O., pp. 725–734. Amsterdam: Elsevier/North-Holland.
18 Keller, E. (1981). In *Progress in Oculomotor Research*, ed. Fuchs, A.F. and Becker, W., pp. 57–62. New York: Elsevier/North Holland.
19 King, W.M. and Fuchs, A.F. (1979). *J. Neurophysiol.* **42**, 861–876.
20 King, W.M., Lisberger, S.G., and Fuchs, A.F. (1986). *J. Neurophysiol.* **56**, 769–784.
21 Luschei, E.S. and Fuchs, A.F. (1972). *J. Neurophysiol.* **55**, 445–461.
22 McElligott, J.G. and Gochin, P.M. (1986). Abstract, Int. Cong. Physiol. Sci. Satellite Meeting, Salishan, Oregon.
23 McElligott, J.G. and Keller, E.L. (1982). In *Functional Basis of Ocular Motility Disorders*, ed. Lennerstrand, G., Zee, D.S., and Keller, E.L., pp. 453–461. Oxford: Pergamon.
24 McIlwain, J.T. (1975). *J. Neurophysiol.* **38**, 219–230.
25 Optican, L.M. and Robinson, D.A. (1980). *J. Neurophysiol.* **44**, 1058–1075.
26 Raybourn, M.S. and Keller, E.L. (1977). *J. Neurophysiol.* **40**, 861–878.
27 Ritchie, L. (1976). *J. Neurophysiol.* **40**, 861–878.
28 Robinson, D.A. (1964). *J. Physiol. (London)* **174**, 245–264.
29 Robinson, D.A. (1970). *J. Neurophysiol.* **33**, 393–404.
30 Robinson, D.A. (1975). In *Basic Mechanisms of Ocular Motility and Their Clinical Implications*, ed. Lennerstrand, G. and Bach-y-Rita, P., pp. 337–374. Oxford: Pergamon.
31 Robinson, D.A. (1981). In *Models of Oculomotor Behavior and Control*, ed. Zuber, B.L., pp. 21–42. Boca Raton: CRC Press, Inc.
32 Rohrer, W.H., White, J.M., and Sparks, D.L. (1987). *Soc. Neurosci.* Abstr. **13**, 1092.

33 Schiller, P.H. (1970). *Exp. Brain Res.* **10**, 347–362.
34 Schiller, P.H. and Koerner, F. (1971). *J. Neurophysiol.* **34**, 920–936.
35 Schiller, P.H., True, S.D., and Conway, J.L. (1980). *J. Neurophysiol.* **44**, 1175–1189.
36 Scudder, C.A. (1986). *J. Neurophysiol.* **59**, 1455–1475.
37 Segravcs, M.A. and Goldberg, M.E. (1984). *Soc. Neurosci.* Abstr. **10**, 389.
38 Sparks, D.L. (1986). *Physiol. Rev.* **66**, 118–171.
39 Sparks, D.L. and Mays, L.E. (1980). *Brain Res.* **190**, 39–50.
40 Sparks, D.L., Holland, R., and Guthrie, B.L. (1976) *Brain Res.* **113**, 21–34.
41 Tweed, D. and Vilis, T. (1985). *Biol. Cybern.* **52**, 219–227.
42 van Gisbergen, J.A.M., Robinson, D.A., and Gielen, S.A. (1981). *J. Neurophysiol.* **45**, 417–442.
43 Waitzman, D. (1982). Ph.D. Thesis, City University of New York.
44 Wurtz, R.H. and Goldberg, M.E. (1972). *J. Neurophysiol.* **35**, 575–586.

12

RELATION OF CORTICAL AREAS MT AND MST TO SMOOTH PURSUIT EYE MOVEMENTS

HIDEHIKO KOMATSU*[1] AND ROBERT H. WURTZ*[2]

Neuroscience Section, Electrotechnical Laboratory, Tsukuba, Ibaraki 305, Japan[1] and Laboratory of Sensorimotor Research, National Eye Institute, National Institutes of Health, Bethesda, Maryland 20892, U.S.A.*[2]*

Pursuit eye movements depend critically on normal motion information processing. This particular type of eye movement acts to keep a moving target on the fovea by matching eye movement to target motion. During pursuit, incomplete matching of eye movement to target motion gives rise to a number of error signals, such as a position error, a velocity error and an acceleration error. Behavioral studies have indicated that the velocity error is the most important of these for generating a smooth eye velocity (*6*).

Several pieces of evidence indicate that the cerebral cortex is important in the generation of pursuit eye movements. In human patients, lesions in the parieto-occipital cortex produce a deficit in pursuit eye movements. In monkeys, two sets of observations have suggested that cells in the superior temporal sulcus (STS), located at the junction between the parietal and the occipital cortices, play a role in the generation of pursuit eye movements. One is the activity of single neurons during pursuit. Sakata and his collaborators found cells in the depth of the STS that discharged during pursuit of a moving target (*11*). To exclude the possibility that activation of the cell resulted from motion of the visual background on the retina during pursuit, they conducted their experiments in a space that was totally darkened except for a lighted target. The second line of evidence is the identification of areas in the STS related to visual motion processing. In recent years, anatomical and physiological studies have established the existence of two serially connected areas in the STS that are devoted to visual motion information processing. One of these areas, the middle temporal area (MT), is located deep on the posterior bank of the STS, and receives a direct projection from layer IVb of the primary visual cortex (the striate cortex or V1) and the thick stripes of area 18 (V2) (see ref. *7*). MT has a high concentration of cells with a direction selectivity to moving visual stimulus. MT in turn projects to the medial superior temporal area (MST), which is located anterior and adjacent to MT on the anterior bank to the fundus of the STS. MST also has a high proportion of the directionally selective cells.

I. PURSUIT CELLS IN MT AND MST

The first direct evidence for the relevance of MT to pursuit eye movements came from the work of Newsome *et al.* (*8*). They made punctate chemical lesions by injecting ibotenic acid into the subarea of MT representing the extrafoveal visual field, and tested the effect on pursuit and saccadic eye movements. They found a deficit in pursuit initiation when the target started to move in the part of the visual field represented by the ablated MT. There was no deficit in the maintenance of pursuit nor in saccadic eye movements made to stationary targets. The recording of neuronal activity from the extrafoveal representation of MT gave results consistent with the lesion study. The cells were activated when the target started to move within their receptive fields and in the same direction as the preferred direction of the cells. However, when the monkey made a saccade in order to bring the fovea near the target, the cells no longer continued to discharge because the target was outside the receptive field. Once the target was brought near the fovea, visual stimulation occurred only around the fovea. Therefore, during the maintenance of pursuit, it is likely that the neurons whose receptive fields include the fovea are activated. We have found this to be true for neurons in MT and MST* that discharged during the maintenance of pursuit (*3*).

A subset of visually responsive cells within the STS was identified as pursuit cells: those cells that discharge during smooth pursuit of a small target in an otherwise dark room. Figure 1 shows examples of such pursuit cells. The left column of Fig. 1 shows the response of a cell recorded from MT. This cell had a small visual receptive field that included the fovea and preferred upward motion. The cell responded during upward pursuit (A) but showed no response during downward pursuit (B). The right column of Fig. 1 shows responses of a cell recorded from MST. This cell had a large receptive field including the fovea, and showed a directionally selective response during leftward pursuit (D and E). As can be seen, the size of the receptive field was quite variable among the pursuit cells, but almost all pursuit cells had receptive fields that included the fovea and showed directionally selective visual responses.

Figure 2A schematically shows the localization of the pursuit cells in MT and MST. Pursuit cells were found only in localized regions: in the foveal region of MT (MTf), in a dorsal-medial area of MST on the anterior banks of the STS that we designated as MSTd, and in a lateral-anterior area of MST on the floor of the STS that we designated as MSTl. As a result of mapping the visual receptive fields in these areas, we have identified several representation of the visual field, which were clear in MT and crude in MST. The lateral part of MT represented the fovea, and in the more medial part, the receptive field became larger and more eccentric. In MST, the cells located at the lateral one-third and the medial one-third both included the fovea in their receptive fields, but the central region represented only the peripheral visual field. Therefore, MTf, MSTd, and MSTl all corresponded to the subareas of MT and MST where the fovea was represented.

*MST was originally defined anatomically by Maunsell and Van Essen (1983) as an area in the STS receiving a projection from MT. However, Desimone and Ungerleider (1986) redefined MST neurophysiologically as a subarea of the projection zone of MT that has directionally selective cells, and we followed this functional definition. See ref. *3* for details.

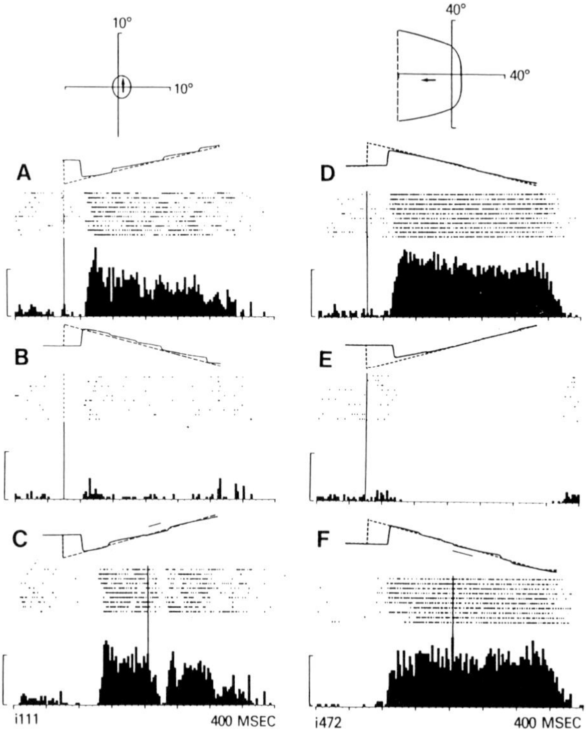

Fig. 1. Examples of two pursuit cells, one recorded from MT (left column) and the other from MST (right column). The drawing at the top of each column is the visual receptive field of each cell. Arrows indicate the preferred direction for stimulus motion. A and D: response during pursuit in the preferred direction. The target stepped downward and moved upward (A) or stepped rightward and moved leftward (D). The target step was 20 deg and the speed of motion was 15 deg/sec. The position traces above the raster illustrate target position (dashed line) and eye position (solid line) for 1 trial. Rasters and histograms are aligned at the onset of the target step. The bin width of the histogram is 20 msec; the ordinate scale is 250 spikes/sec/trial. B and E: response of these cells during pursuit in the null direction. C and F: effect of blink of the target during pursuit in the preferred direction. The blink of the target for 150 msec is indicated by the solid line along the position trace; the rasters and histograms are aligned at the point of the blink. (Adapted from ref. *9*)

II. ORIGIN OF PURSUIT DISCHARGE IN MT AND MST

The distribution of pursuit cells in MT and MST seems to agree with the hypothesis that the activity of these cells during pursuit originat-

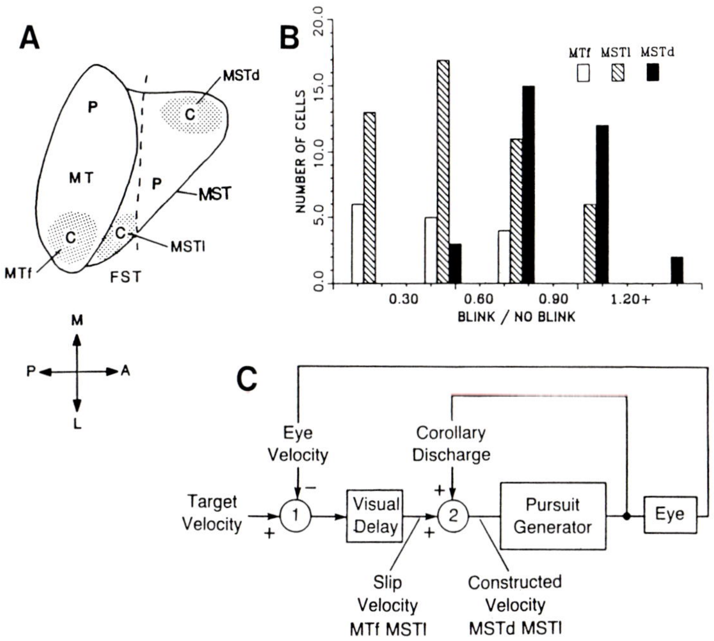

Fig. 2. A: localization of pursuit cells in MT and MST. Shaded areas represent subareas where pursuit cells were found. Within MT and MST, "C" indicates areas representing the central visual field, and "P" indicates areas representing the peripheral visual field. The dashed line denotes the fundus of the STS. Arrows indicate anterior (A)-posterior (P) directions, and medial (M)-lateral (L) directions. B: ratio of the pursuit response during target blink to the response without blink. Cells are in the 0.3-unit-wide bins. C: block diagram summarizing the possible functional relationship among MTf, MSTd, and MSTl cells in relation to the generation of pursuit eye movements. (Adapted from refs. *3* and *9*)

ed from the visual stimulation by the target around the fovea. However, the discharge during pursuit could result either from this visual stimulation by the target motion on the retina (retinal velocity slip) or from some other input such as an extraretinal input related to the pursuit movement itself. We tested the relative importance of each of these possible inputs by removing the visual motion stimulus during pursuit either by blinking off the visual target briefly or by stabilizing the target on the retina (*9*). To stabilize the target on the retina, the eye position signal was used to drive a mirror galvanometer which controlled the target position. If a cell was driven by the retinl slip of the target, its activity should decrease with this reduction in target motion. Pursuit cells in MTf clearly decreased their rate of discharge during blink or stabilization of the target, indicating that they were mainly driven by the retinal velocity slip of the target. The cell in the left column of Fig. 1 is an example of such a cell. Figure 1C shows the effect of blink of the target. Although the eye movement itself did not change clarly during blink (short bar under the eye trace), the activity of the cell clearly decreased. On the other hand, pursuit cells in MSTd continued to discharge during pursuit despite blink or stabilization of the pursuit target, indicating that they were mainly driven by an extraretinal input. An example of such a cell is shown in the right column of Fig. 1. In MSTl, some cells were like those of MTf, others were like those of MSTd. Figure 2B summarizes the effects of the blinking off of the target in MTf, MSTd, and MSTl.

We also observed a relationship between pursuit responses and passive visual responses: cells whose pursuit responses were attributable to visual inputs tended to prefer well-localized simuli such as small spots, and cells whose pursuit responses were attributable to extraretinal inputs tended to respond preferentially to large-field random dot patterns.

The characteristics of the pursuit cells in MTf described above were consistent with the notion that they were encoding the velocity error signal. This was also the case for some of the pursuit cells in MSTl. As this is an important signal for maintaining pursuit, an effect on the eye velocity can be expected to result from a change in the neuronal activities in these area. Dürsteler *et al.* (*1*) and Dürsteler and Wurtz (*2*) elimnated the activity of cells in MT and MST by creating punctate chemical lesions, and observed a decrease in eye velocity during the maintenance of pursuit when the lesion was made either in MTf or in MSTl. But such an effect was not observed when a lesion was made in MSTd. This deficit was a directional one: only pursuit toward the side of the lesion was affected. We recently examined the effect of electrical stimulation (50–150 μA) on pursuit eye movements throughout areas MT and MST (*5*). An acceleration toward the side of the stimulation occurred when the stimulation was applied to MTf or MSTl, but there was no consistent effect when MSTd was stimulated. Therefore, these lesion and stimulation experiments have also supported the notion that the velocity error signal carried by cells in MTf or MST1 was likely to be used to drive smooth pursuit. So far, there have been no data which could explain the directionality of the effect.

Although the retinal velocity error is an important signal for maintaining pursuit, a subject can maintain eye velocity in the absence of this signal, such as during afterimage tracking. To explain this, a model in which a corollary of eye velocity is added to the retinal slip velocity to construct the target velocity in space has been proposed (*12*). Such a constructed velocity could drive the pursuit generator even in the absence of any retinal velocity slip. The pursuit cells observed in MST that are driven by an extraretinal input are possible candidates for carrying the constructed velocity signal, and Fig. 2C illustrates this. Careful measurements of the latency of the extraretinal input in these pursuit cells showed that they were not active until after the onset of the pursuit; this is consistent with the idea that the extraretinal input to these cells is a corollary discharge of the command for the pursuit. However, the visual input to many of these pursuit cells in MST responds optimally or exclusively to large-field random dots, and this makes it unlikely that the cells encode the constructed velocity. Only a minority of the cells in MST1 remain candidates for carrying the constructed velocity signal, because they receive an extraretinal input and prefer small spots as a visual stimulus.

III. MST AND PERCEPTION

Pursuit eye movements are usually made to follow a target moving over a visual background. As a result of the pursuit movement, this background is moved across the retina and should also activate the motion-sensitive pursuit cells. We have examined the visual response to large-field motion of pursuit cells in MT and MST, and the influence of the background on the pursuit response (*4*). All the pursuit cells in MTf and some in MST1 responded preferentially or at least equally well to small spots as compared to large-field stimuli. The effect of the visual background on the pursuit response in these cells was relatively weak. The remaining pursuit cells in MST1 and almost all pursit cells in MSTd responded preferentially to large-field motion, and in these cells, a significant interaction of the visual background with the pursuit response was frequently observed. Over three-fourths of these cells showed a preferred direction of the visual response to large-field motion that was opposite to the pursuit response. For example, a cell that responded to rightward motion of a random dot pattern during fixation responded best during leftward pursuit made in the dark. For many of these cells, the pursuit response was driven mainly by an extraretinal input. As can be expected from the relationship between the preferred directions, about 85% of such cells showed a pursuit response in the light that was enhanced compared to that in the dark.

The significance of such an enhancement on pursuit is not clear because behavioral data have shown that there is little influence on or a slight degradation in the maintenance of pursuit made against a lighted background, as compared to that made in the dark. One possible function of this enhancement in relation to pursuit might be to compensate for the optokinetic nystagmus potentially produced by the large field stimulus moving in the direction opposite to that of the pursuit. Anothr possibility is that these cells are related more to the perception of motion than to the generation of pursuit.

There is a parallel relationship between the conditions under which these pursuit cells discharge and our perception of motion of a small spot occurs: one is during pursuit of a target in one direction, and the other is during fixation of a stationary spot with motion of a large field in the opposite direction. During pursuit eye movements, even if there is no retinal slip, as is the case in afterimage tracking, we still clearly perceive motion of the target in the same direction as that of the pursuit. This is presumably due to an extraretinal input, and these pursuit cells receive such extraretinal input. When a large field is moving in the background during fixation of a stationary spot, our perception is that the spot is moving in a direction opposite to that of the large-field motion. These pursuit cells respond to large-field motion in a direction opposite to the preferred direction of the pursuit response. There is another condition under which we perceive motion of a small stimulus in the same direction as above: when a small stimulus moves in that direction while we are fixating on a stationary spot. We observed that the discharge and the perception were parallel in this condition as well for many of these pursuit cells.

We found that, in many of these cells, the visual response showed a reversal of the preferred direction of motion as the size of the stimulus field changed. When the field size was small, the preferred direction of the visual response was the same as that of the pursuit response, while, when the field size was large, they were opposite each other. Figure 3A gives an example. When a monkey was fixating on a stationary spot (FP), we presented five different sizes of moving random dots fields. When the field size was small (10 to 20 deg on an edge), downward movement of the dots produced a stronger response than the upward movement. However, when the field size was large (40 or 73 deg on an edge), the preferred direction was reversed and the upward movement produced a stronger discharge than the downward movement. A possible explanation for this reversal is that the receptive field of the cell had a central and a peripheral area with opposite preferred directions, as shown schematically in Fig. 3B. If this were the case, such a cell would be more likely to be important in detecting the local contrast of the direction in the velocity field. However, this possibility was rejected as a result of the experiment illustrated in Fig. 3C. The preferred direction of the small field of random dots was always the same, regardless of the location of presentation within the 40 deg square, although the stimulation of the entire 40 deg field showed the opposite preferred direction. This indicates that the difference in the spatial summation properties of the two directions is likely to be responsible for the reversal.

Figure 3D schematically shows the suggested mechanism for the reversal of the preferred direction. For the cell shown here, the activation of each local area of the field by an upward motion is fed to an AND gate, so that the activation is conveyed as an output of this cell only when the entire field is stimulated. On the other hand, the activation by downward motion of each local area of the field is fed to an exclusive OR gate, so that the activity is relayed to the output only when the stimulation is a local one. Therefore, these pursuit cells have properties that satisfy the expectations for cells related to a perception of motion that is independent of the retinal event: visual responses to small stimuli moving in one direction

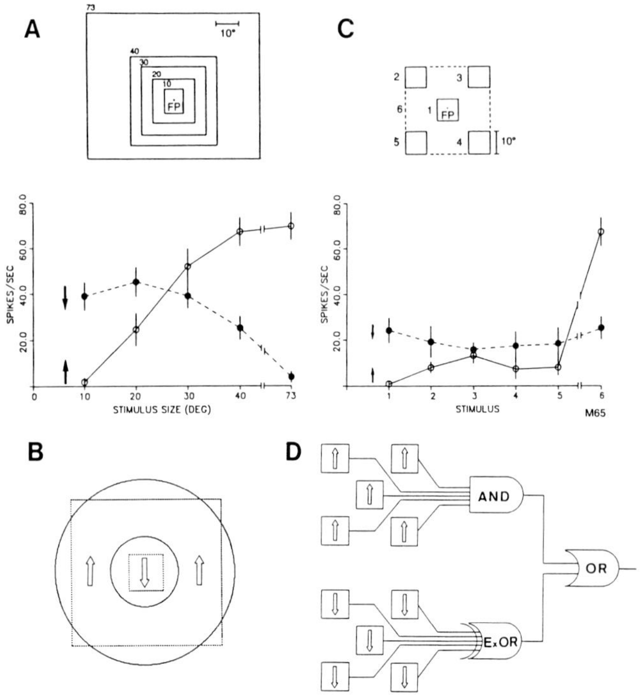

Fig. 3. An example of a cell showing a reversal of the preferred direction with an increase in stimulus size, and models of the receptive field to explain this reversal. A: at the top is a schematic illustration of the five sizes of random-dot fields used. The number above each rectangle indicates the square root of the area of the random-dot field. FP is the fixation spot. At the bottom is a graph of the relationship between the size of the dot field and the magnitude of response. Directions of stimulus motion are indicated by arrows. B: a schematic illustration of a receptive field having an organization in which the preferred directions (arrows) of the central and surrounding subfields (circles) are opposite each other. The random-dot fields located at appropriate places (squares) can explain the reversal of the preferred direction observed in A. C: effect of motion of a 10 deg random-dot pattern at different locations (1–5) or of a 40 deg field (6) on the same cell as in A. The different positions of the small stimulus did not lead to a reversal of the response, only the larger stimulus (6) did, refuting the prediction from the model shown in B. D: a schematic illustration of a spatial summation property that explains the results of C. Squares correspond to the locations 1 to 5 of the random-dot field in C. The effects of the upward and downward directions of motion are shown separately. (A and C are adapted from ref. *4*.)

pursuit-related responses due to an extraretinal input in the same direction, and visual responses to large-field motion in the opposite direction.

Another possible function related to perception is one more relevant to body movements than to eye movements. While pursuit eye movements produce movement of the entire visual field in the same direction and at the same speed, body movements produce a motion parallax that can result in heterogeneous velocity fields, depending on the configuration of the environment. If the subject sways his body from right to left while fixating on a stationary object in space, his eyes move in a direction opposite to that of body movement. At the same time, a stimulus located between the subject and the fixated object moves across the retina in a direction opposite to that of body movement, whereas a stimulus located further away from the fixated object moves in the direction of body movement. Therefore, these pursuit cells carry the kinds of signals included in this situation, and they can be regarded as carrying useful information about the depth of the objects located in the environment. This possibility of the depth perception involving body movement is particularly interesting in relation to cells in MSTd. Saito *et al.* have reported that in the dorsal half of MST (which probably corresponds to MSTd), many cells respond to change in size or rotation of visual stimuli (*10*). These modes of stimulus motion obviously have a close relation with such body movements as locomotion or tilting in the frontal plane. Although there is as yet no behavioral evidence of this, MSTd may be important in analyzing visual motion information resulting from body movements. On the other hand, there is clear evidence that MSTl plays a role in the maintenance of pursuit. If this area is also related to some aspect of perception, it seems more reasonable to assume that it is the consequence of pursuit eye movement, not body movement, that MSTl is monitoring.

SUMMARY

We recorded neuronal activity from motion-related areas in the STS of the monkey. We investigated both the visual properties of neurons and their response during smooth pursuit eye movements, a behavior that is critically dependent on visual motion processing. In MT, the first stage of motion processing in the STS, visual activation of the cells by the retinal velocity error of the target was observed during pursuit. In MST, a stage of visual processing following MT, a divergence in the visual and oculomotor characteristics was evident. Cells preferentially responding to small spots were driven by the retinal velocity error of the target during the pursuit, and may provide the visual signal required to generate the pursuit. Other cells that preferred large-field motion tended to receive extraretinal input as well. These cells integrate visual and pursuit-related inputs and may indicate the perceptual consequences of the pursuit.

REFERENCES

1 Dürsteler, M.R., Wurtz, R.H., and Newsome, W.T. (1987). *J. Neurophysiol.* **57**, 1262–1287.
2 Dürsteler, M.R. and Wurtz, R.H.(1988). *J. Neurophysiol.* **60**, 940–965.
3 Komatsu, H. and Wurtz, R.H. (1988). *J. Neurophysiol.* **60**, 580–603.
4 Komatsu, H. and Wurtz, R.H. (1988). *J. Neurophysiol.* **60**, 621–644.
5 Komatsu, H. and Wurtz, R.H. (1989). *J. Neurophysiol.*, in press.
6 Lisberger, S.G., Morris, E.J., and Tychsen, L. (1987). *Annu. Res. Neurosci.* **10**, 97–129.
7 Maunsell, J.H.R. and Newsome, W.T. (1987). *Annu. Rev. Neurosci.* **10**, 363–401.
8 Newsome, W.T., Wurtz, R.H., Dürsteler, M.R., and Mikami, A. (1985) *J. Neurosci.* **5**, 825–840.
9 Newsome, W.T., Wurtz, R.H., and Komatsu, H. (1988). *J. Neurophysiol.* **60**, 604–620.
10 Saito, H.-A., Yukie, M., Tanaka, K., Hikosaka, K., Fukada, Y., and Iwai, E. (1986). *J. Neurosci.* **6**, 145–157.
11 Sakata, H., Shibutani, H., and Kawano, K. (1983). *J. Neurophysiol.* **49**, 1364–1380.
12 Yasui, S. and Young, L.R. (1975). *Science* **190**, 906–908.

13

HOW IS THE VISUAL ASSOCIATIVE MEMORY REPRESENTED IN NEURONS OF THE PRIMATE TEMPORAL CORTEX?

YASUSHI MIYASHITA, KUNIYOSHI SAKAI, AND SEI-ICHI HIGUCHI

Department of Physiology, Faculty of Medicine, University of Tokyo, Tokyo 113, Japan

I. WHERE IS THE MEMORY STOREHOUSE?

The visual memory function, subserving the identification of objects, has been assigned to the multisynaptic occipito-temporo-limbic projection (*9*) which interconnects the striate, prestriate, inferior temporal, and hippocampal cortices (Fig. 1). Physical properties of a visual object (such as its size, color, texture, and shape) are analyzed in the multiple subdivisions of the prestriate-posterior temporal complex (*21*). The anterior part of the inferior temporal cortex (area TE, according to Bonin and Bailey) is hypothesized not only to synthesize the analyzed attributes into a unique configuration but also to work as the storehouse for central representations of the objects, since damage of this area affects visual recognition of objects in humans (*6*) and monkeys (*8*). Damage of the hippocampus and/or related parahippocampal cortices also impairs object recognition (*22, 23*), but is accompanied by only a short-span retrograde amnesia (*7, 22*), suggesting that the hippocampal system does not work as the

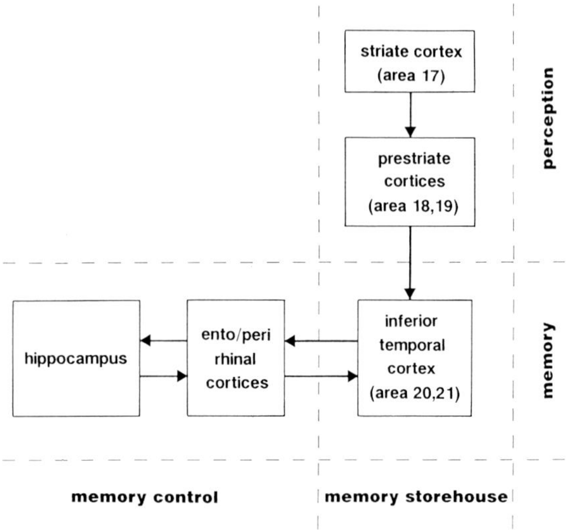

Fig. 1. A hypothetical view of the functional structure of the visual memory system.

memory storehouse, but instead as the machinery controlling the memory processes (Fig. 1).

However, single-unit recordings from the anterior temporal cortex have been unsuccessful in identifying the neuronal correlate of the visual memory traces. Some neurons fire selectively to specific complex objects, including hands and faces (*2*), but the discharges cease soon after offset of the stimulus presentation, leaving uncertainty as to whether any of these neurons could serve the short-term memory of complex objects. It has not been tested whether the selectivity of these neural responses is innately determined, or developed during the early critical period (as in some neurons in the striate cortex), or acquired through learning during adulthood, thus also leaving it open whether any of these neurons could serve the pictorial long-term memory.

Recently, we found a neuronal correlate (*10*, *12*, *13*) of the visual memory storehouse as predicted by the hypothesis outlined in Fig. 1. The neurons were characterized both by activation while the subjects (monkeys) memorized a stimulus in the working memory, and by acquired stimulus-selectivity through learning. In this article we

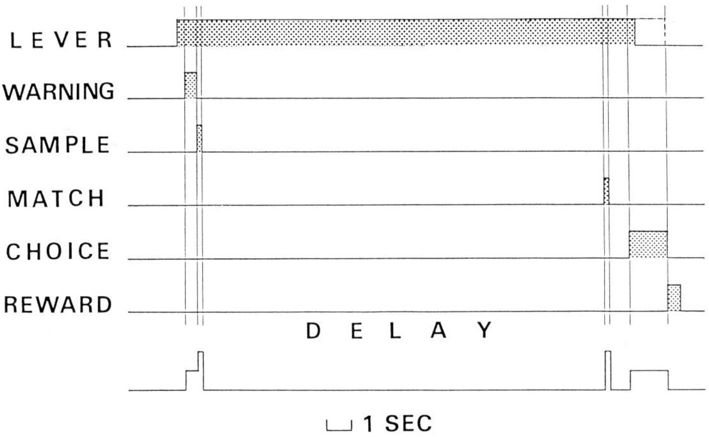

Fig. 2. Sequence of events in a trial. LEVER, lever press by the monkey. WARNING, warning green image. SAMPLE, sample stimulus. MATCH, match stimulus following a 16 sec delay. CHOICE, choice signal of white image. Bottom trace, events-chart used in Figs. 3, 4, 6, and 7.

review the characteristics of these memory neurons and discuss how they fit in with the schema of Fig. 1.

II. BEHAVIORAL TASK AND RECORDING OF NEURAL ACTIVITIES

In a trial of our visual memory task (delayed matching-to-sample task), sample and match stimuli were successively presented on a video monitor, each for 0.2 sec at a 16 sec delay interval (Fig. 2). Three adult monkeys (*Macaca fuscata*) were trained to memorize the sample stimulus during a delay period and then to decide whether the match stimulus was the same as the sample. A correct response was rewarded with fruit juice. A set of 97 color patterns was generated by a fractal algorithm with a 32-bit seed of random numbers (*11*); the set was repeatedly used during an over-training session ("learned stimuli") in a fixed sequence according to an arbitrary attached number (serial position number, SPN). While extracellular discharges of a neuron were recorded (*14*), a sample stimulus was selected not only from the 97 learned patterns but also from a new set of 97 patterns ("new stimuli"). Different sets of new stimuli were created for each neuron using the same algorithm but a different seed. The

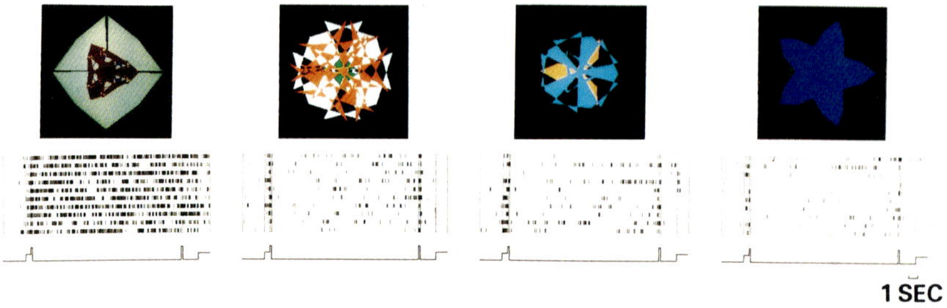

(Fig. 3)

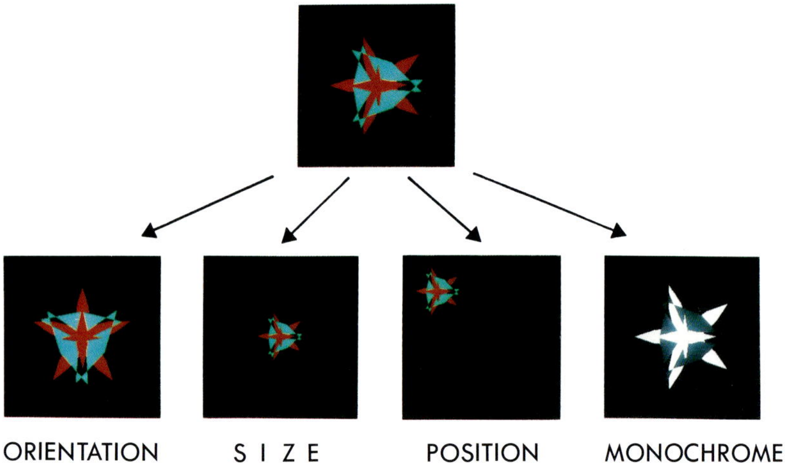

(Fig. 5)

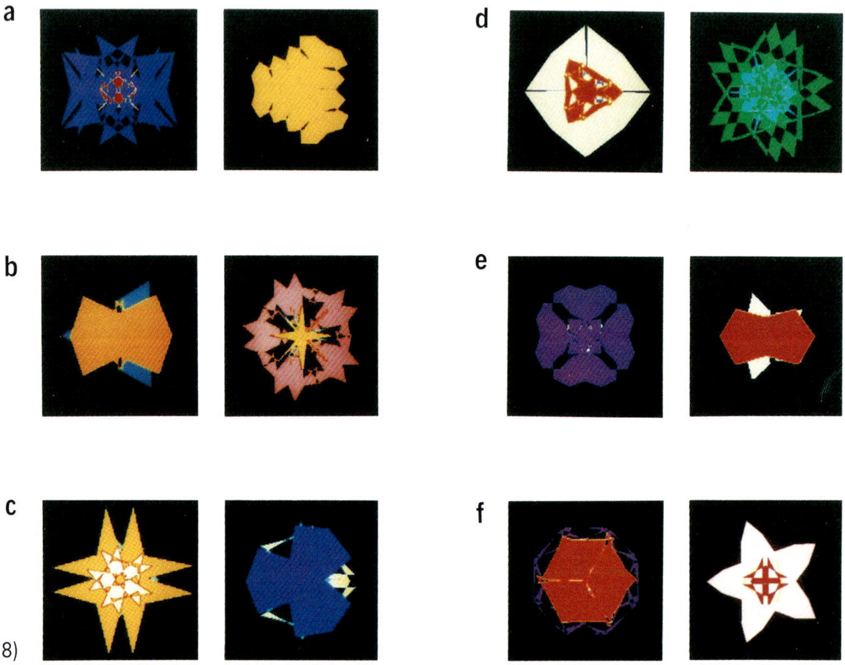

(Fig. 8)

learned stimuli and new stimuli were used at random, independent of the SPNs.

III. NEURAL DISCHARGES RELATED TO THE WORKING MEMORY

A few of the 97 learned stimuli reproducibly activated a particular neuron with high-frequency sustained discharges during the delay period of the task. Figure 3 illustrates one representative cell for 4 different sample stimuli (prominent in a, but virtually ineffective in b, c, and d). A time course of the delay activity in Fig. 3a is shown as a spike density histogram (Bin width, 200 msec) in Fig. 4, as contrasted with those for 6 other ineffective stimuli. It is notable that the optimal picture differed from cell to cell, and that the entire population of the optimal pictures for the tested cells covered a substantial part of the repertory of the pictorial stimuli.

IV. CATEGORIZED PERCEPT OF A PICTURE IS MEMORIZED

For further analysis of triggering features of the delay responses, sample pictures were manipulated in the following manner (Fig. 5): 1) stimulus size was reduced by half, 2) stimuli were rotated by 90 degrees in a clockwise direction, 3) colored stimuli were transformed into monochrome by referring to a pseudo-color look-up table, and 4) stimulus position was changed on the video monitor (a 0.2 sec stimulus presentation time is short enough to exclude the contribution of saccadic eye movement). Figure 6 illustrates responses of a neuron which consistently fired during the delay after one particular picture but not after others, irrespective of stimulus size (Fig. 6Ab, Bb), orientation (Fig. 6Ac, Bc), or color (Fig. 6Ad, Bd). Similar

---

←Fig. 3. Stimulus selectivity of delay discharges. Spike discharges of a cell are shown in cases when the monkey memorizes different fractal patterns. Each rastergram consists of trials whose sample stimulus is shown above. Trials of the same sample stimulus were originally separated by intervening trials of other sample stimuli, and these were sorted and collected by off-line computation.

Fig. 5. Transformations of visual stimuli.

Fig. 8. Colored fractal patterns which produced the strongest and second strongest delay discharges in learned stimuli for 6 different cells (a-f). Note that the two optimal stimuli for a neuron have no similarities in their geometric patterns.

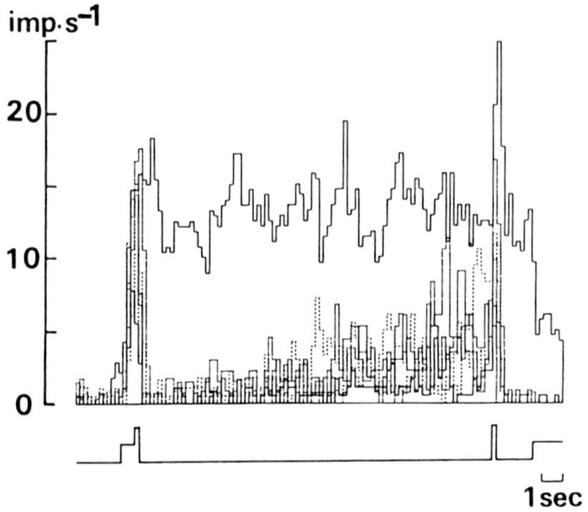

Fig. 4. Time-course of delay discharges. Spike density histograms for trials with different sample stimuli were superposed. Bin width, 200 msec.

tolerance of responses was observed in a majority of the tested delay neurons: to size in 16/19, to orientation in 5/7, to color-monochrome in 15/20, and to position in 8/13 cells. In other neurons, manipulation of the most effective stimulus reduced or abolished the thereby-evoked delay discharge.

V. STIMULUS-SELECTIVITY IS ACQUIRED THROUGH LEARNING

A few of the 97 learned stimuli were effective in activating high-frequency sustained delay discharges in a cell (Fig. 7a, b). By contrast, 97 new patterns produced only weak delay responses (Fig. 7c, d). The distribution of the delay discharge rate to the new stimuli (Fig. 7d) lacked the small population of high-frequency responses (>2 impulses/sec) which characterized the distribution to the learned stimuli (Fig. 7b).

Of the 206 neurons recorded in the anterior ventral temporal cortex of the over-trained monkeys, 57 neurons exhibited shape-selective delay discharges, and 17 of the 57 cells were successfully tested with both learned and new stimuli. In these 17 cells, the maximum delay discharge for learned stimuli (arrow in Fig. 7b) was always larger than that for new stimuli (arrow in Fig. 7d), and the

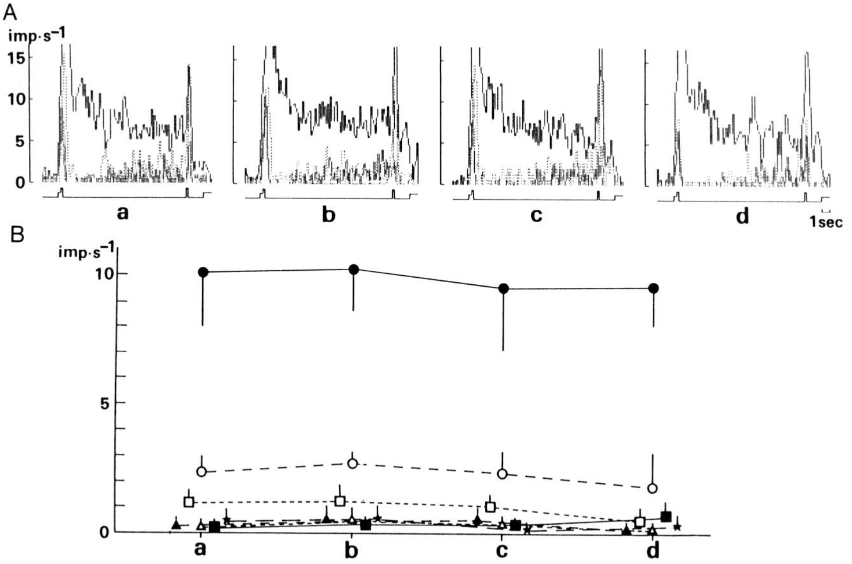

Fig. 6. Response tolerance under stimulus transformation in size, orientation or color. A: histograms similar to Fig. 4, but for 5 different sample pictures. (a), control responses. (b), (c), and (d) show the effects of stimulus size reduction by half, stimulus rotation by 90 degrees in a clockwise direction, and color-to-monochrome transformation. B: average delay spike frequencies as a function of stimulus transformation (a, original; b, size reduction; c, rotation; d, color to monochrome). Responses to 7 different sample pictures (including 5 shown in A) are plotted with different symbols. Error bars indicate standard deviations for 4–15 trials.

difference was highly significant ($p<0.001$, Wilcoxon test). When the selectivity of a neuron to a set of 97 patters was represented by the sharpness of the response distribution (the kurtosis of the distribution (*17*), the selectivity to the learned patterns was almost always (15/17) higher than that to the new patterns ($p<0.005$). In spite of the presence of a few effective pictures in the learned stimuli, there was no difference between the median response to the learned and new stimuli (double arrows in Fig. 7b, d) for the 17 cells ($p>0.5$). These results suggest that the sharpness of the response selectivity of these neurons to the learned patterns was formed throughout the course of training.

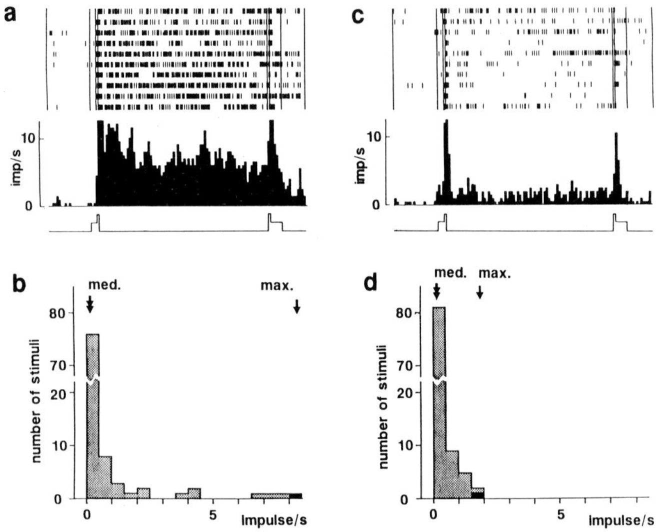

Fig. 7. Neural activity to the "learned" and "new" stimuli. a: raster recordings of impulse discharges and spike density histogram obtained from a cell in trials where a "learned" picture was used as a sample stimulus. b: frequency distribution of the average firing rate measured during the delay period following 97 "learned" sample pictures in the same cell. The black column indicates the response shown in Fig. 7a. ↓ max. and ↓ med., maximum and median value in the distribution. c, d: similar illustration to a and b but "new" pictures are used as sample stimuli in the same cell. The black column in d represents the response illustrated in Fig. 7c.

VI. ACQUIRED SELECTIVITY REPRESENTS THE ASSOCIATIVE LONG-TERM MEMORY

In human long-term memory, ideas and concepts become associated through learning. Is it possible that the training determines not only how sharply the effective learned patterns are represented in each neuron (as shown above) but also which patterns are conjointly chosen as the few optimal stimuli? I first examined the geometric similarity of the optimal stmuli of a cell, and found that the stimuli were often completely different, as seen in Fig. 8 for 6 cells, suggesting a non-geometric criterion in choosing these patterns as the optimal stimuli of a cell. I then examined the effect of a fixed-order presentation of the patterns during the training session according to an

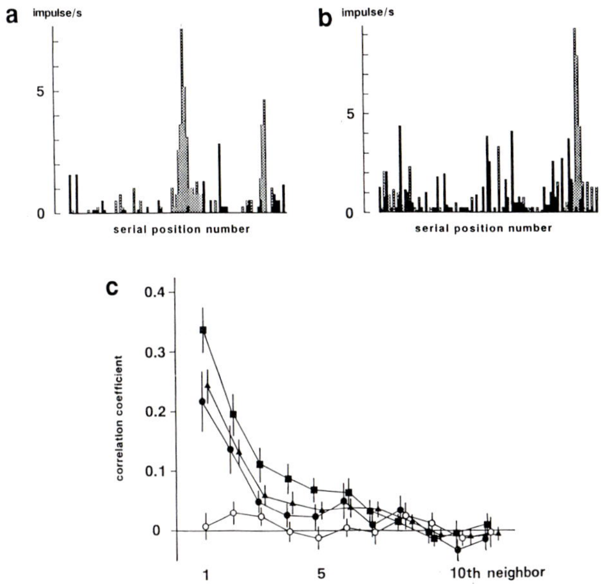

Fig. 9. Stimulus-stimulus association among the learned fractal patterns. a: average delay discharge rate (impulse/sec) for each sample stimulus in a cell. Abscissa, SPN of the sitmuli. Stippled columns, learned stimuli. Black columns, new stimuli. b: same as a, for a different cell. c: autocorrelograms of the delay discharge rate along the SPN of the stimuli. ● and ○, average autocorrelogram for the learned and new stimuli in the 17 cells. ▲, that for the learned stimuli in the 57 cells. ■, that for the learned stimuli in the 28 cells for which the nearest-neighbor correlation along the SPN was significant ($p<0.05$) according to Kendall's test. Error bars, standrd errors. ***: $p<0.001$, **: $p<0.01$, *$p<0.05$, according to the Kolmogorov-Smirnov test in comparison with the value for new stimuli.

arbitrarily attached SPN. If the consecutively presented patterns tended to be associated together, and if the association was fixed in the choice of effective patterns for a cell, we could expect to find the effective patterns correlated along the SPN, in spite of a random presentation of the stimuli during the unit-recording session.

Figure 9a and b shows for 2 neurons that the effective responses to the learned stimuli indeed cluster along the SPNs (stippled columns). The clustering was not due to an artifact in the testing procedure because the responses simultaneously obtained from the new stimuli were not clustered (black columns). In the 17 cells which were tested with both learned and new stimuli, the responses to the learned stimuli were significantly correlated (Fig. 9c, ●) in the nearest-neighbor of the SPNs, as compared with the responses to the new stimuli (○) ($p<0.01$, Kolmogorov-Smirmov test). The 57 cells tested by the learned stimuli exhibited similar correlated responses along the SPN (▲). The nearest-neighbor correlation for the learned stimuli differed from cell to cell, and was significant ($p<0.05$) in 28 of the 57 cells according to Kendall's correlation test (*17*), while that for the new stimuli was not significant in any of the 17 cells.

VII. COMPARISON WITH OTHER TEMPORAL CORTICAL NEURONS

In the primate inferior temporal (IT) cortex, neural discharges selective to specific complex objects have been reported (*2*), such as for hands, face, and Fourier descriptors. However, the selectivity of these sensory responses appeared to be organized along the patterns' geometrical similarity. The present neurons were selective to the artificial fractal patterns and had two distinct properties compared to other shape-selective IT neurons: first, the present neurons were active in the delay period of the working-memory task, that is, when the visual stimulus was off and the monkey memorized it. Second, most of the other sensory neurons were located posterior to the presently explored area, TE_{av} (*18*) (or TE_1-TE_2 (*16*)). The TE_{av} has been anatomically designated as the last link from the visual system to the limbic memory systems (*3*, *8*, *19*), especially the hippocampus (*20*). Thus, we propose that this interaction with the limbic system plays a key role in organizing neuronal selectivity for the association of geometrically dissimilar pictures, as illustrated in Fig. 1.

VIII. NEURAL REPRESENTATION OF THE MEMORY STOREHOUSE

The discovery of these pictorial neurons not only supports the schema shown in Fig. 1. but also gives more concrete, vivid shape to the neural representation of the visual memory storehouse.

Firstly, pictorial short-term memory is coded by temporary activation of an ensemble of neurons in the visual association cortex (*2*), rather than by neuronal activity in a brain area specialized for short-term memory. Although each neuron in the ensemble has highly abstract and selective coding features, representation of the memory of a picture seems to be distributed among a number of neurons.

Secondly, a cognitive model for memory assumes that ideas in the working memory are the activated elements in the associative long-term memory (*1*). The present results fit well with such a model, since the effects of learning upon stimulus-stimulus association are revealed in the neurons which represent the working memory of the categorized percept of pictures (*10*, *12*).

Thirdly, we have directly shown that the responses of a single IT neuron reflect an experimentally-controlled association between a temporally related set of stimuli. There are indirect clues indicating the occurrence of such association during daily life; in the polysensory areas deep within the superior temporal sulcus (mainly, area TPO), which receive a projection from the IT cortex (*4*), some cells were selective for a person's different perspective views (face or body movement) (*15*), which might be interpreted by an associative experience between the perspective views that are visually distinct but temporally related in many occasions. Visual associative agnosia (*5*) in humans may result from selective loss of the neurons thereby encoding the association between visually dissimilar objects.

SUMMARY

A hypothetical functional diagram on the primate visual memory system is proposed in which the inferotemporal cortex (area TE) is considered as the memory storehouse. To test this hypothesis, single-unit activities of the temporal cortical neurons were examined while the monkeys were performing a visual memory task (delayed matching-to-sample (DMS) task). We found shape-selective neurons that exhibited sustained activity during the delay period of the DMS task. The activity was highly selective for the pictorial information to be memorized and was independent of the physical attributes such as size, orientation, color or position of the object, suggesting that the delay activity represents the short-term memory of the categorized percept of a picture. Moreover, the selectivity of these delay discharges developed through repeated trials of the DMS task. Computer-generated artificial patterns were used as the stimuli to be memorized. The few patterns for which a neuron was conjointly selective were frequently related to each other through stimulus-stimulus association imposed during the course of training. Thus,the selectivity acquired by these cells is suggested to represent the associative long-term memory of pictures. These observations not only support the proposed hypothesis but also give more concrete, vivid shape to the neural representation of the presumed memory storehouse.

Acknowledgments
This work was supported by grants from the Yamada Foundation and from the Japanese Ministry of Education, Science and Culture (63870007).

REFERENCES

1 Anderson, J.R. and Bower, G.H. (1980). Human Associative Memory. Hillsdale, New Jersey: Lawrence Erlbaum Publ.
2 Gross, C.G. (1972). In *Handbook of Sensory Physiology*, vol. VIII/3B, ed. Jung, R., pp. 451–482. Berlin: Springer-Verlag.
3 Herzog, A.G. and Van Hoesen, G.W. (1976). *Brain Res.* **115**, 57–69.
4 Jones, E.G. and Powell, T.P.S. (1970). *Brain* **93**, 793–820.
5 McCarthy, R.A. and Warrigton, E.K. (1986). *J. Neurol. Neurosurg. Psych.* **49**, 1233–1240.
6 Milner, B. (1968). *Neuropsychologia* **6**, 191–209.
7 Milner, B., Corkin, S., and Teuber, H.L. (1968). *Neuropsychologia* **6**, 215–234.
8 Mishkin, M. (1982). *Phil. Trans. R. Soc. Lond., Ser. B* **298**, 85–95.
9 Mishkin, M., Ungerleider, L.G., and Macko, K.A. (1983). *Trends Neurosci.* **6**, 414–417.
10 Miyashita, Y. (1988). *Nature* **335**, 817–820.
11 Miyashita, Y. (1988). In *Dynamic Interactions in Neural Networks: Models and Data*, ed. Arbib, M.A. and Amari, S., pp. 183–192. Berlin: Springer-Verlag.
12 Miyashita, Y. and Chang, H.S. (1988). *Nature* **331**, 68–70.
13 Miyashita, Y., Cho, K., and Mori, K. (1987). *Soc. Neurosci.* Abstr. **13**, 608.
14 Miyashita, Y. and Nagao, S. (1984). *J. Physiol.* **351**, 251–262.
15 Perret, D.I., Mistlin, A.J., and Chitty, A.J. (1987). *Trends Neurosci.* **10**, 358–364.
16 Seltzer, B. and Pandya, D.N. (1978). *Brain Res.* **149**, 1–24.
17 Snedecor, G.W. and Corcoran, W.G. (1980). *Statistical Method*. Iowa: Iowa

University Press.
18 Turner, B.H., Mishkin, M., and Knapp, M.J. (1980). *Comp. Neurol.* **191**, 515-543.
19 Van Hoesen, G.W. and Pandya, D.N. (1975). *Brain Res.* **95**, 1-24.
20 Yukie, M. (1988). *Neurosci. Res.* (Suppl.) **7**, S16.
21 Zeki, S. and Shipp, S. (1988). *Nature* **335**, 311-317.
22 Zola-Morgan, S., Squire, L.R., and Amaral, D.G. (1986). *J. Neurosci.* **6**, 2950-2967.
23 Zola-Morgan, S., Squire, L.R., and Amaral, D.G. (1988). *Soc. Neurosci.* Abstr. **14**, 1043.

PROGRAMMING IN NEURONAL NETWORK AND SYSTEM

14

NETWORK MODELS FOR EYE MOVEMENT CONTROL

MASAHIKO FUJITA

Communications Research Laboratory, Ministry of Posts and Telecommunications, Tokyo 184, Japan

In an early study Pitts and McCulloch (*5*) outlined a theoretical network model of the superior colliculus (SC) which can generate oblique saccades. At that time, little was known about the brain stem organization of eye movements. With the accumulation of research on this topic, we are now able to discuss the mechanism involved in oblique saccade generation.

Robinson (*8*) proposed a saccadic control system essentially as a position-servo system with local feedback. A new local feedback model, proposed by Scudder (*9*), contains the SC output signal as a motor command and demonstrates a good simulation of neural signals in the brain stem.

The SC is a motor center of the saccade system in the brain stem. A well-defined retinotopic map of the contralateral visual field is formed in the SC in which the central visual field is represented anteriorly, and the peripheral visual field posteriorly. The upper fields are represented medially, and the lower fields laterally. The visual map also functions as a motor map of sacades (Fig. 1); collicular stimulation in the deeper layers evokes a saccade to a point in the visual space from which the superfical layer unit, just superior

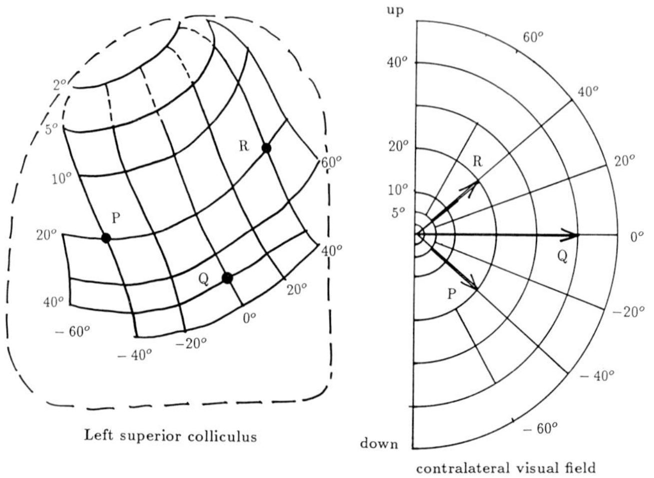

Fig. 1. The motor map formed on the SC (after Robinson, *7*). Stimulation at sites P, Q, and R in the left SC evoke corresponding and respective saccades P, Q, and R to the contralateral visual field.

to the stimulation site, has received visual input until the initiation of the saccade (*7, 12*).

All of this research has been directed at how to reveal the neural mechanism of spatial-to-temporal transformation; visual or spatial information of the gaze shift in specific amplitude and direction must be transformed into corresponding temporal signals of oculomotor neurons. Such spatial-to-temporal transformation can be explained by constructing neural network models for the superior colliculus, the nerve fiber projection to the reticular formations and the premotor neuron circuits.

I. POPULATION CODING MODEL OF THE SACCADE

1. A Simple Principle

In Fig. 2 the nerve fibers are projected in parallel to a neuron pool. When an input signal traverses the central fibers of the tract, it will activate many dendrites in the neuron pool, and the total activity of this pool will increase. Inversely, an input signal along the more peripheral fibers of the tract will cause less activity in the neuron pool. The total amount of activity depends on the location of the

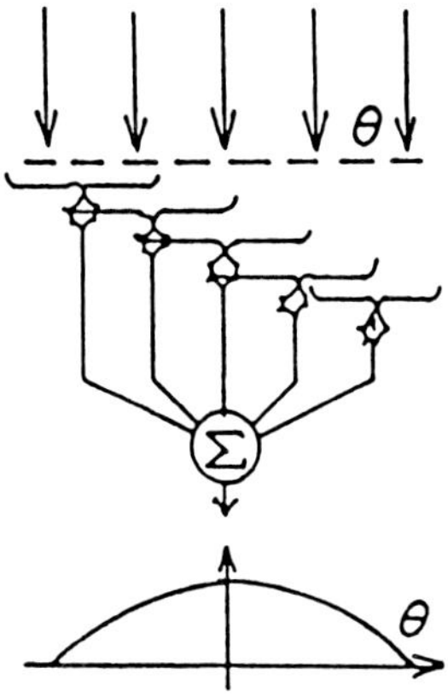

Fig. 2. A simple principle of population coding. Total amount of activity of a neuron pool depends on the active site (θ) of the input fibers.

input signal, as shown in the lower part of Fig. 2. Taking the highest value at the middle, and assigning a value of 0 to both ends, a convex function of the transformation resembles a trigonometric cosine function.

When the strength of the input signal changes, the total activity will change accordingly. Assuming linearity in the input-output relationship of the neurons, we obtain the total amount of activity as the product of the input signal strength and a value of the trigonometric cosine-like function. This principle constitutes a neural basis of spatiotemporal transformation in the present model. We presume that the neuron pool would consists of long-lead burst neurons (LLBNs) which receive direct input from the SC.

2. A Hypothesis of Nerve Fiber Projection from the SC to the Premotor Neurons

Collicular outputs activate premotor neurons in the brain stem. A hypothesis of nerve fiber projection from the SC to four LLBN pools, shown in Fig. 3, accounts for the generation of oblique saccades. For generating a horizontal component of a saccade, the SC projects output fibers into a contralateral LLBN pool. For a vertical component, both medial halves of the SCs project fibers side by side into another LLBN pool to generate an upward component of saccades.

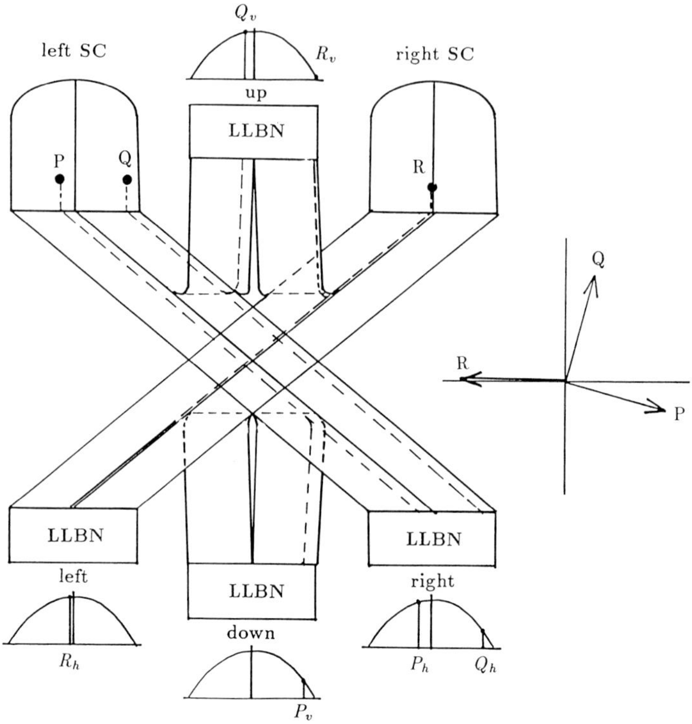

Fig. 3. Hypothetical nerve fiber projection from the SC to four burst neuron pools (LLBNs). Collicular stimulation at P generates a horizontal and vertical component of the saccade as P_h and P_v, respectively, according to the principle of population coding (Fig. 2).

Descending nerve fiber bundles from the lateral halves of both SCs first cross each other, and then travel in parallel into another LLBN pool to generate a downward component of saccades. By these projections and the population coding principle in the former section, the horizontal and vertical components become proportional to $\cos(\theta)$ and $\sin(\theta)$, respectively, where θ denotes the saccade direction. We presume that LLBNs mediate signals from the SC to these burst neuron pools.

3. Hypotheses of the Saccade Amplitude Coding

Collicular output units seem to have identical activity patterns (*11*). This leads us to the postulation that the number of output units or descending fibers involved in generating a saccade determines the amplitude. Regarding the amplitude coding, some hypotheses have been presented by physiologists along this line (discussion summary by Fuchs, *1*). The hypotheses on which the present model is based, with some modifications, are described in section II-1.

II. A PROPOSED SYSTEM OF INHIBITION IN THE SC

1. Circuit

We assumed the following four groups of saccade-related neurons, designated by O_1, O_2, O_3, and I layers in the SC (Fig. 4).

1) The final output units of the SC are differentially distributed in the O_1 layer. The unit density is proportional to the saccade amplitude which the location of the unit encodes. Each dendrite of the neurons covers a circular area of a definite size.

2) Units are uniformly distributed in the O_2 layer. They excite the neighboring units within a circular area of a defnite radius, ρ.

3) The units in the O_2 layer activate not only the O_1 layer units, but also the O_3 units and I units. The O_3 units are excitatory, and activated by signals from diverse brain areas. They discharge at a constant rate, and activate the pause neurons (PNs) in the pons.

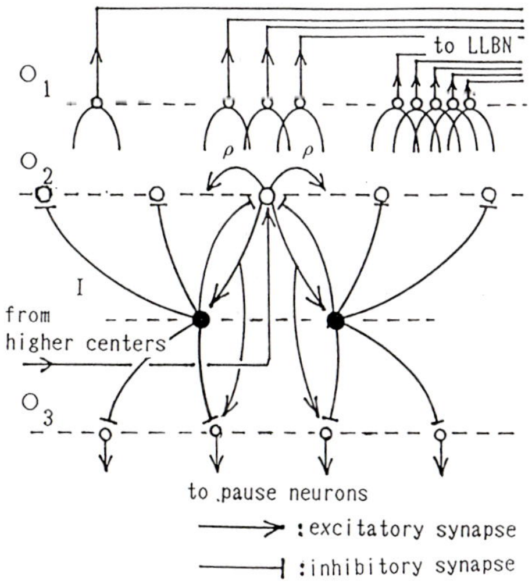

Fig. 4. A proposed system of inhibiton in the output layers of the SC.

4) The I units have a powerful inhibitory effect. Their inhibitory actions occur bilaterally on all units in the O_3 layer, as well as reciprocally on all units in the O_2 layer.

An alternate version of (1) can be described as follows: (1′) The final output units of the SC are uniformly distributed in the O_1 layer. The unit at a particular location has axon collaterals, the number of which is proportional to the saccade amplitude encoded by the location of the unit.

When collicular stimulation is strong enough, the PNs cease firing for 20 msec (*6*). The present model proposes that this type of inhibition is also due to the function of the I layer in suppressing the excitatory O_3 units.

2. Spatial Interaction of Collicular Stimulations at Two Sites

Simultaneous stimulation at two sites in the SC evokes a single saccade, which is not a sum but a weighted mean of the two saccades which result when each site is self-stimulated (*7*). The above model of the SC accounts for the neural excitation process in the O_2 layer in the following way: activated by a motor signal from higher centers (FEF or SNr; ref. *13*), some neurons in the O_2 layer initiate burst discharge. The excitation spreads, consecutively activating neighboring units in the O_2 layer. Each unit at the excitation front is activated by the units behind within a distance of ρ. The total intensity of the activation remains constant. Excitation in the O_2 layer will b e accompanied by the activation of the I units with some delay. Suppressive reaction of the I units on the O_2 layer gradually increases in proportion to the size of the active area in the O_2 layer. Eventually, the suppression overcomes the activation, the active area reduces in size and finally disappears (Fig. 5 in ref. *10*).

Let us designate, by S, the maximum size of an activated circular area in the O_2 layer when the suppression and activation are balanced. The activation intensity in the front units is a function of ρ, and the suppression intensity is a function of S. We designate them by $E(\rho)$ and I(S), respectively. Then it holds that $E(\rho)=I(S)$.

Let us consider the case when two different sites in the SC initiate the process of excitation simultaneously. If two areas, S_1 and S_2, are in the equilibrium state (Fig. 5), the total suppression intensity

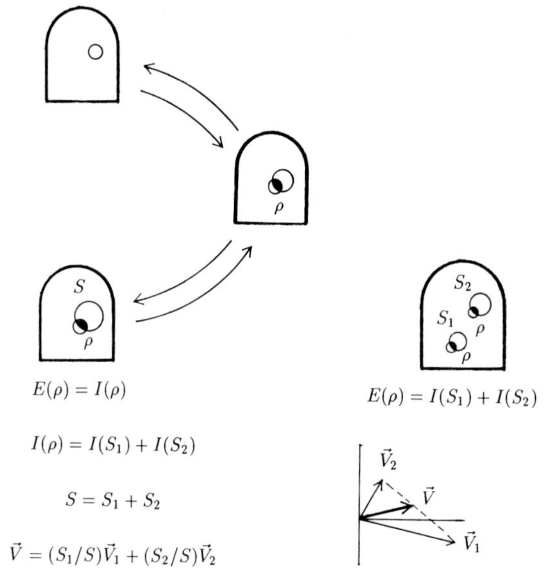

Fig. 5. Calculated result of a model of spatial interaction of saccades simultaneously evoked by two stimuli in the SC.

becomes a combination of $I(S_1)$ and $I(S_2)$, which balances with $E(\rho)$; it thus holds that $E(\rho)=I(S_1)+I(S_2)$, and then $I(S)=I(S_1)+I(S_2)$. If we assume linearity of the function I(S), then $S=S_1+S_2$. The number of units in excitation at S_1 or S_2 is reduced to the ratios S_1/S and S_2/S. Let the saccade vector, determined by the site S_1 or S_2, be V_1 or V_2, then the evoked saccade V by simultaneous stimulations at S_1 and S_2 becomes $V=(S_1/S)V_1+(S_2/S)V_2$, according to the theory of population coding of oblique saccades (*2–4*).

SUMMARY

A motor command, encoded spatially in the SC, is transformed to temporal patterns of motor neuron excitation in the brain stem. Such spatial-to-temporal transformation is explained by constructing neural network models for the SC, nerve fiber projection to the reticular formations and premotor neuron circuits.

The SC is assumed to have a reciprocal inhibition system in the output layers, as well as a differential distribution of the final output units whose density is proportional to the amplitude of a spatially coded saccade. Thus, the SC can encode the amplitude of a saccade as the number of output units in the excitation.

The excitation signals generate horizontal and vertical components of the saccade through the hypothesis of specific nerve fiber projection from the SC to burst neurons in the brain stem. Topological consideration of these projections leads to the expected generation of two-dimensional elements of an oblique saccade by population decoding of the LLBNs, based on the principle that a neuron pool will excite the greater part as an input signal enters the more central part of the pool.

REFERENCES

1 Fuchs, A.F. (1981). In *Progress in Oculomotor Research*, ed. Fuchs, A.F. and Becker, W., pp. 115–121. New York: Elsevier/North-Holland.
2 Fujita, M. (1987). US-Japan Joint Seminar "Competition and Cooperation in Neural Nets 2" at USC, Los Angeles.
3 Fujita, M. (1988). Population coding of two-dimensional saccades in the brain stem. INNS First Annual Meeting, Boston.
4 Fujita, M. (1988). A proposed system of inhibition in the deeper layers of the superior colliculus. INNS First Annual Meeting, Boston.
5 Pitts, W. and McCulloch, W.S. (1947). *Bull. Math. Biophys.* **9**, 127–147.
6 Raybourn, M.S. and Keller, E.L. (1977). *J. Neurophysiol.* **40**, 861–878.
7 Robinson, D.A. (1972). *Vision Res.* **121**, 1795–1808.
8 Robinson, D.A. (1975). In *Basic Mechanisms of Ocular Motility and Their Clinical Implications*, ed. Bach-y-Rita, P. and Lennerstrand, G., pp. 337–374. Oxford: Pergamon.
9 Scudder, C. (1984). *Soc. Neurosci.* Abstr. **10**(2), 910.
10 Sparks, D.L., Holland, R., and Guthrie, B.L. (1976). *Brain Res.* **113**, 21–34.
11 Sparks, D.L. and Mays, L.E. (1980). *Brain Res.* **190**, 39–50.
12 Sparks, D.L. (1986). *Physiol. Rev.* **66**, 118–171.
13 Wurtz, R.H. and Hikosaka, O. (1986). *Prog. Brain Res.* **64**, 175–190.

15

NEURAL NETWORKS FOR GENERATION OF EYE AND ARM MOVEMENT TRAJECTORIES

ROLF ECKMILLER

Department of Biophysics, University of Düsseldorf, D-4000 Düsseldorf 1, Federal Republic of Germany

The most prominent output of the various information processing events in the brain is represented by continuous signal time functions to control the various motor systems (*e.g.*, eye-, speech-, or arm movements). Thereby the brain continuously generates movement trajectories, namely spatio-temporal events.

Biological motor systems are typically redundant (with more degrees of freedom than necessary for the desired types of movement), nonlinear, and non-orthogonal systems. Obviously nature can deal with such parallel, asynchronous, redundant, and nonlinear motor systems. Novel technologies for implementing networks with many thousands of processing elements (neurons), distributed memory elements (synapses), and flexible network topology offer the opportunity to overcome some major obstacles towards building brain-like (of course, at a very primitive level) machines for motor control (*1*, *10*).

I. ARTIFICIAL NEURAL NETWORKS FOR MOTOR CONTROL IN INTELLIGENT ROBOTS

Biological motor control systems for rhythmic time functions such as those controlling heartbeat, locomotion, and respiration (*11*, *19*) are assumed to be based on a small number of neurons. In these cases the time parameter is represented by oscillations and time constants of neural activity within a small neural net that is capable of internally generating the required time functions even without sensory feedback from muscles or joints.

For quasi-ballistic goal directed movements (*e.g.*, reaching, pointing, saccadic eye movements), various mathematical and neural models have been proposed to explain the typical correlation between amplitude, velocity profile, and duration of the movement (*2*, *4*, *5*, *12–14*).

A quite different kind of neural motor program generator is required for non-rhythmic and non-ballistic smooth movements such as speech movements, voluntary limb movements (dancing, drawing, or gesticulating), or pursuit eye movements. Biological data on neural networks that act as function generators for such smooth movement trajectories are scarce (*3*, *6*, *17*, *20*).

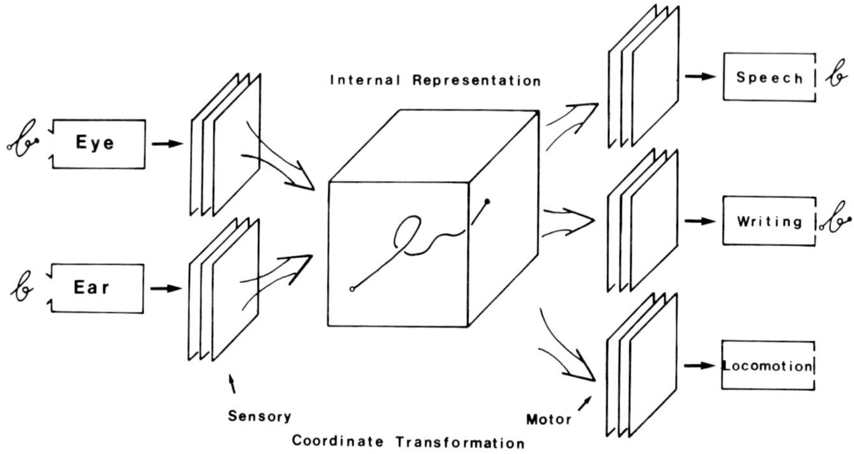

Fig. 1. Scheme of an intelligent robot as a federation of various neural net modules.

The vertebrate central nervous system with its many distinct brain regions can be considered to be a federation of 'special purpose' neural nets (*e.g.*, visual cortex, cerebellum). Intelligent robots (Fig. 1) are currently being conceived and designed that consist of various neural net modules with special purpose functions such as: a) pattern recognition, b) associative memory, c) internal representation of patterns and trajectories, d) generation of motor programs, and e) sensory as well as motor coordinate transformation (*8*). The blocks eye and ear in Fig. 1 represent modules for visual and auditory trajectory detection (not necessarily including pattern recognition). Both sensory input modules receive signal time courses, which occur as spatiotemporal trajectories at the level of the corresponding sensory receptor array (retina or basilar membrane in vertebrates). The vision module, for example, monitors the event of a letter 'b' being written by a teacher, whereas the hearing module is thought to monitor the acoustic event of a spoken 'b'.

It is assumed here that each sensory module is connected with the internal representation module *via* a specific sensory coordinate transformation module (depicted as a three-layered structure). The function of these coordinate transformation modules is to map a given sensory trajectory onto a normalized trajectory to be stored in the internal representation module. For the sake of simplicity we might think of these internally stored trajectories as paths in the 3-dimensional space of a neural net, along which a particle or neural activity peak can travel with constant or varying speed. The internal representation module can store very large amounts of different trajectories, which could share neural elements.

The subsequent generation of a corresponding movement trajectory (Fig. 1) for drawing a letter 'b' or speaking a 'b' is assumed here to require the activation of the appropriate stored desired trajectory. Please note that pattern recognition is not required for these sensorimotor tasks. In fact, the pattern recognition process might operate on the basis of the internally stored trajectories, which are available for iterative recognition procedures after the end of the sensory event. For the purpose of motor program generation, an activity peak (see below and ref. 7) travels along the stored path on the neural net of the internal representation module.

The desired trajectory can be thought of as the 2-dimensional trajectory of the fingertips while drawing the 'b', or as the virtual center of contraction of all speech muscles while vocalizing a 'b'.

In redundant motor systems such as for arm- or speech movements specific motor coordinate transformation modules serve to transform the internally generated desired trajectory into a set of simultaneous control signals for the individual actuators (motors, muscles).

The schema of an intelligent robot in Fig. 1 emphasizes the notion that large portions of information processing in both animals and robots with neural net control involve *handling of spatiotemporal trajectories* for the purpose of detection, recognition, storage, generation, and mapping. It is proposed that the time parameter in these 'trajectory handling neural nets' is not defined by a central clock but is implicitly represented by the propagation velocity of neural activity peaks within the neural net.

II. FUNCTION GENERATOR FOR DESIRED MOVEMENT TRAJECTORIES

The generation of non-rhythmic and non-ballistic smooth velocity time courses requires a flexible neural net acting as a function generator. A neural net model (7) for internal representation and generation of 2-dimensional movement trajectories including pursuit eye movements is described below (Fig. 2). This model accounts for sensory updating, prediction, and storage, and it is biologically (at least in principle) plausible though not based on experimental data. The key features of this neural function generator can be summarized as follows:

1) The velocity time course in one movement direction is represented by the trajectory of a neural activity peak (AP) that travels with constant velocity from neuron to neuron.

2) The neural net is arranged as a neural triangular lattice (NTL) on a circular surface.

3) The triangular lattice output signal is proportional to the eccentricity of the activity peak relative to the center.

NTL topology: consider a large number of identical processing elements (neurons) with analog features. These neurons are arranged

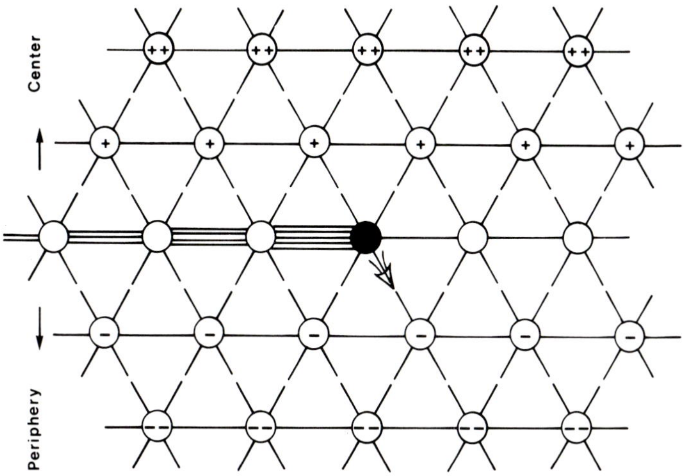

Fig. 2. NTL with a travelling AP as neural net for generation and storage of various movement velocity functions.

in a NTL, in which they are connected only to their 6 immediate neighbors. Such a triangular lattice with a radius of 50 neurons from the center to its periphery would consist of about 8,000 neurons. The connectivity strength c_T of tangential synaptic connections between neurons located along concentric circles about the center is slightly larger than c_R for synapses of radial connections. Each neuron has a subthreshold potential P similar to the membrane potential of biological neurons. The potential is always assumed to represent the average of the potential values of all immediately neighboring neurons due to continuous equilibration of possible potential gradients *via* neural connections. External potential changes can only be applied to the NTL center, thus yielding a center-symmetrical potential field. Such an input-dependent potential field can be thought of as an elastic circular membrane whose center is being pushed up or down.

NTL dynamics: a suprathreshold AP can be initiated (or extinguished) only at the center, and becomes superimposed on the potential field. For the sake of simplicity, the AP can be thought of as a neural action potential (*18*) or a soliton (*15*), which travels away from the center (following the potential field gradient during a positive potential input) in the same angular direction (3 o'clock) upon its initiation at the center.

AP travels with constant propagation velocity from one neuron to one of its neighbors, and its activity does not otherwise spread. Every time the activity peak arrives at a neuron, a decision has to be made concerning its next destination. Due to certain transient constraints imposed on the adjacent synapses by the travelling AP, only those 3 of the 6 neighboring neurons can be selected that are located in forward (straight, right, or left) continuation of the trajectory. The decision as to which of the 3 possible target neurons is selected is based on a combined evaluation of the connectivity strength c and the potential gradient dP/dR between the neighboring neurons.

If the potential field P is flat throughout the NTL, the AP will select the tangentially adjacent neuron, since the connectivity c_T is slightly larger than c_R for radial connections. In the case of a positive potential input at the center, however, the potential field exhibits a radial gradient towards the periphery, which in effect pulls the activity peak towards the periphery (equivalent to higher velocities at the triangular lattice output). Similarly, a negative input attracts the AP towards the center.

A portion of the triangular latticer together with the AP (filled circle) and the last portion of the memory trace of its trajectory is shown in Fig. 2. Horizontal connections in Fig. 2 are assumed to follow circles about the center. The AP had travelled from the left and is about to move towards the NTL periphery due to an assumed sudden positive potential step input at the center.

A memory trace of the most recently traversed portion of the trajectory is created by means of a temporary increase of the connectivity strengh as indicated by the number of connecting lines in Fig. 2. It is assumed that the memory trace, which gradually fades with a time constant of about 1 sec, serves as a trajectory guide for subsequent movements, for example, during post-pursuit eye movements after sudden target disappearance and for neural prediction during pursuit of a periodically moving target.

III. LEARNING AND RETRIEVAL OF DESIRED MOVEMENT TRAJECTORIES

The detailed synaptic connectivity pattern of 3 adjacent lattice neurons is shown in Fig. 3 to describe the topology of an element of this triangular lattice. The neurons (large open circles with axon-like projections and synapses) are reciprocally connected *via* the synapses. Two additional neurons with pre-synaptic synapses (synapse on another synapse), a pattern retrieval (PR) neuron and a velocity modulation (VM) neuron have contacts with the triangular lattice. The PR neuron belongs to a large population of identical PR neurons for storage and retrieval of entire trajectories that always begin and end in the NTL-center. It is assumed that each PR neuron has excitatory synapses (small circles) on each of the synapses. In contrast, the VM neuron has inhibitory synapses (depicted as open blocks) on each of the triangular lattice synapses in order to control the propagation velocity v of the AP on the triangular lattice.

When a given trajectory has to be learned (stored), while being generated by means of input modulation of the potential field, one of the PR neurons (that had not been used before) is first selected for this task, as indicated by the big arrow.

In the present example it is assumed that the AP travels along

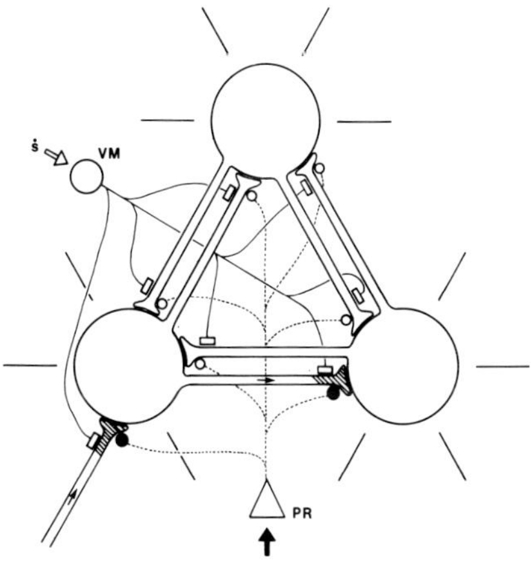

Fig. 3. Neural net topology of three adjacent NTL neurons together with a PR neuron and a VM neuron.

a given trajectory (from bottom left to right) including the two hatched lattice synapses in Fig. 3. The connectivity strength of those few synapses which belong to the selected PR neuron and have a pre-synaptic connection with the lattice synapses along the AP trajectory (here, the two hatched synapses) becomes permanently increased. This process is assumed here to represent learning (memory) and is indicated by an enlargement of the two corresponding PR synapses (filled circles). The weighting factors of the other pre-synaptic synapses as well as of all synapses of the non-selected PR neurons remain low (except for those synapses that were involved in storing other trajectories). In this way a single PR neuron stores one trajectory during the process of its first generation on the NTL. The later retrieval of this permanently stored trajectory is implemented by a brief activation pulse for the corresponding PR neuron. This activation pulse is assumed to yield a strong temporary enhancement of those NTL synapses that compose the desired trajectory, thus creating a memory trace. Immediately afterwards the AP becomes initiated in the lattice center. AP travels (although the potential input to the NTL center is zero) along this temporarily existing memory trace as in the groove of a record. Again, the triangular lattice output monitors the radial AP distance during constant propagation velocity of AP and thereby generates the previously stored velocity time function R(t) proportional to $\dot{s}(t)$. This model contains elements of the engram hypothesis (*16*).

IV. NEURAL NET MECHANISMS FOR GEOMETRIC REPRESENTATION OF ROBOT ARM KINEMATICS

As indicated in Fig. 1, it is proposed here to partition the neural net system for the motor control of an intelligent robot into two modules: A) a neural space net for internal representation of external space including obstacles and of desired movement trajectories in real time, and B) a neural kinematics net for kinematics representation and transformation or mapping of desired movement trajectories to a set of simultaneous control signal time courses for the actuators of the redundant robot in real time. Whereas the NTL model (Figs. 2 and 3) is suggested to serve as neural space net, a novel concept for the

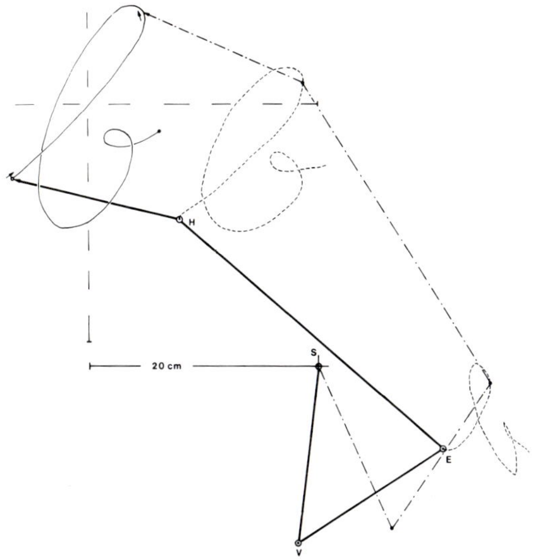

Fig. 4. Scheme of a 4-joint machine for generation of horizontal trajectories. The b-shaped trajectories at fingertip (arrow), hand joint (H), and elbow joint (E) indicate a typical human arm movement.

neural kinematics net is described below. As test bed for a redundant robot system a 4-joint machine (*9*) is proposed for the simulation of horizontal arm movements in an operation plane of 40 cm $\times$ 40 cm, with the vertical projection of the shoulder joint S as stationary center of the reference system. Figure 4 depicts the 4-joint machine with four actuators for rotatory movements about the joints: S (shoulder), V (virtual joint), E (elbow), and H (hand). While fingertip F (arrow) generates a trajectory like the handwritten letter 'b', the interupted paths at joints H and E indicate a typical human arm movement while writing this letter 'b'. The geometric configuration of the 4-joint machine, which is thought to simulate the human arm movement approximately in the horizontal plane, is indicated in Fig. 4 for the starting point of the trajectory and at a later time along the trajectory.

It is assumed here that a desired trajectory (*e.g.*, a 'b' to be written by the machine) has been provided by the neural space net. The goal of the neural kinematics net is to minimize a given cost function (*e.g.*, minimization of both rotation angles e_i relative to the neutral position and their increment Δe_i at all joints i). The geometric

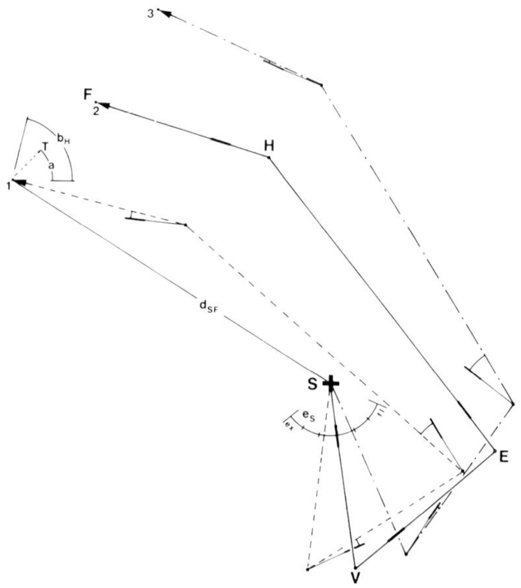

Fig. 5. POM as neural map for continuous monitoring of the geometry of the 4-joint machine.

representation of the inverse kinematics of this 4-joint machine is subdivided into several distinct neural net maps and mechanisms for knowledge representation:

1) The position model (POM) is a neural map which serves for continuous 'book keeping' of the various distances, positions, and angles of the 4-joint machine (Fig. 5). These values are automatically being updated when the 4-joint machine moves fingertip F by a small trajectory element T(a) in the direction of angle a. Each joint has an operation range of 60 deg extension (ex) and 60 deg flexion (fl). Figure 5 depicts the 4-joint geometry for three fingertip positions (1, 2, and 3). In position 2 which forms the center of the operation plane, all four joints are in their neutral positions.

2) The angle model (ANM) is an ensemble of neurons with circular direction characteristics incorporating all horizontal preferred directions. Each joint is represented in ANM by a set of four direction-selective neurons (Fig. 6). The current directions from a given joint to the fingertip F are provided by POM and indicated in Fig. 6, by the arrows d_{HF}, d_{EF}, d_{SF}, and d_{VF}. ANM receives the

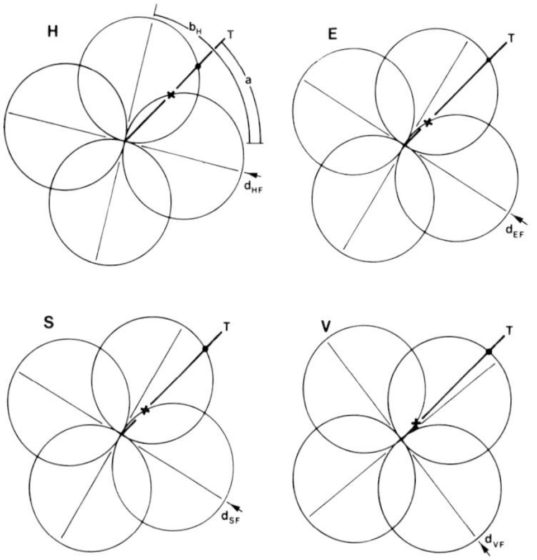

Fig. 6. ANM as a neural ensemble which selects 4 direction-selective neurons (with circular characteristics) for each joint (H, E, V, and S) in order to specify the movement components in the direction of- and orthogonal to- the current trajectory element T(a).

current direction angle a for the desired next trajectory element T(a) as stimulus. Each of the four sets of direction-selective neurons responds with an impulse rate (filled dots) proportional to the movement component of a given joint at F in the desired direction a, as well as with another impulse rate (crosses) proportional to the orthogonal movement component.

3) The contribution selector mechanism (CSM) in Fig. 7 uses the various geometric parameters provided by POM and ANM in order to decide about the contributions of the four individual joints to the current trajectory element T(a). Since the four joints can only generate rotations, they contribute to the movement of fingertip F in characteristic directions (by means of fl or ex).

Assuming that all four joints are moving as little as possible and stay as close as possible to their neutral positions, the angle command mechanism (ACM) uses POM, ANM, and CSM to implement a simple non-iterative procedure, which yields the corresponding movement directions and rotation angles of the four actuators. Please note that this procedure emphasizes geometric operations such as separation of vectors into components and vectorial addition of movement vectors. The first step of ACM is to find the movement vectors C_i at fingertip F as a result of a 1 deg rotation at joint i. In order to enhance the tendency of each joint i to stay close to its neutral position, a gain $G_i(e_i)$ with values between 0 (60 deg excursion in one direction) and 2 (60 deg excursion in the opposite direction) is being defined. $G_i(e_i)=1$ in the neutral position ($e_i=0$).

$$(1) \qquad C_i(mm)=\frac{\pi}{180}\cdot G_i(e_i)\cdot d_i(mm)$$

Figure 7 indicates the various movement vectors C_i at fingertip F (large filled circle) for 1 deg rotations towards ex or fl. ACM finds the geometric vector addition (as shown in Fig. 7) of those C_i vectors which yield a resultant movement vector M as close as possible to the desired trajectory element T(a) with an assumed standard length of 1 mm.

Secondly, ACM adjusts the direction of M to that of T(a). For this purpose, ANM provides the vector components orthogonal to T(a). Figure 7 depicts the positive sum ($sum_{pos.}$) and the negative sum ($sum_{neg.}$) of these orthogonal components. The difference (diff.) between these two sums is subsequently used to find scaling factors P and N for the positive and negative components:

(2) $P\cdot sum_{pos.}-N\cdot sum_{neg.}=0$, is the result of this scaling procedure, which yields the desired directional adjustment.

(3) $P=(sum_{pos.}-diff./2)/sum_{pos.}$;
$N=(sum_{neg.}+diff./2)sum_{neg.}$

This scaling step transforms all C_i into D_i, thus yielding a vectorial addition (filled dot in the direction of T(a) in Fig. 7).

The third step of the angle control mechanism (ACM) serves to adjust the length of D_i by a common scaling factor K so as to reach a vectorial sum of the four D_i vectors equal to the assumed standard length of 1 mm for T(a).

$D_i\cdot K=E_i$, the adjusted movement vectors of the four joints at fingertip F. The corresponding rotation angle increments Δe_i(deg) are given as:

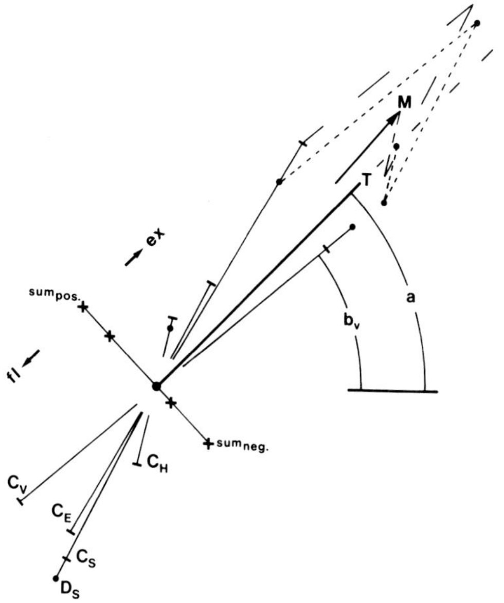

Fig. 7. CSM. CSM finds the appropriate movement vectors for the 4 joints to yield the desired fingertip movement as defined by T(a).

$$\Delta e_i(\text{deg}) = \frac{180}{\pi} \cdot \frac{E_i}{d_i} \tag{4}$$

These proposed neural net mechanisms indicated in Figs. 5–7 are fundamentally different from the classical algebraic-analytical representation of the inverse kinematics of a robot arm, which are typically defined by a large set of differential equations. In this regard, the concept for the neural net control of a 4-joint machine (Fig. 4) could be compared with a smart clockwork with flexible cam disks and gears, which does 'not know' at all times how to move between any two positions in its operation plane. Rather, the clockwork 'knows' precisely how to move a small distance (*e.g.*, the standard length of 1 mm) from its current position P into any possible direction a, and represents most parameters and their relations geometrically rather than algebraically. Although this concept for inverse kinematics representation of a redundant robot arm is not based on specific neurophysiological data and does not (at the present time) include the dynamics of the 4-joint machine, it nevertheless allows emphasis of several important points:

a) Biological neural systems are not known for their ability to solve mathematical problems by algebraic-analytical equations. Instead, the available body of neurobiological data indicates that neurons with their characteristic receptive field properties can be interpreted as geometric measurement and mapping devices, such as eccentricity detectors, direction detectors, Gabor function filters, etc.. Furthermore, the typical topologies of biological neural nets (*e.g.*, retina, visual cortex, or cerebellar cortex) as multi-layered neural maps suggest geometric mapping operations rather than algebraic calculations.

b) Since the presently available digital computers automatically force the scientist to write the program of a given mathematical problem by means of algebraic-analytical equations, research in brain theory and neural programming may benefit from devices such as artificial neural network simulators or neural computers (*1*, *10*) with the ability to process geometric representations of certain classes of mathematical problems (*e.g.*, pattern recognition or robot control).

c) The understanding and development of *neural programs for motor control* in biological and technical motor systems requires not only studies on various learning rules to generate the desired neural net topology by means of self organization, but also research on the geometrical processing power of various neural net topologies defined by intuition and a knowledge of geometry as well as neuroscience.

Acknowledgment

This work was supported by the Federal Ministry for Research and Technology (BMFT).

REFERENCES

1 Anderson, D.Z. (ed.) (1988). *Neural Information Processing Systems.* New York: American Institute of Physics.

2 Arbib, M.A. (1981). In *Handbook of Physiology*, vol. II, ed. Brookhart, J.M., Mountcastle, V.B., and Brooks, V.B., pp. 1449–1480. Baltimore, MD: Williams & Wilkins.

3 Baron, R.J. (1987). In *The Cerebral Computer—An Introduction to the Computational Structure of the Human Brain*, ed. Baron, R.J., pp. 402-452. Hillsdale, New Jersey: Lawrence Erlbaum Publ.
4 Berkinblit, M.B., Feldman, A.G., and Fukson, O.I. (1986). *Behav. Brain Sci.* **9**, 585-638.
5 Eckmiller, R. (1983). *IEEE Trans. on Systems, Man and Cybern.*, vol. 13, pp. 980-989.
6 Eckmiller, R. (1987). *Physiol. Rev.* **67**, 797-857.
7 Eckmiller, R. (1987). *J. Neurosci. Meth.* **21**, 127-138.
8 Eckmiller, R. (1988). In *Neural Computers*, ed. Eckmiller, R. and v.d. Malsburg, C., pp. 359-370. Heidelberg: Springer-Verlag.
9 Eckmiller, R. (1988). *Neural Networks* **1** (Suppl.) 334. Boston: First Annual Meeting International Neural Networks Society.
10 Eckmiller, R. and v.d. Malsburg, C. (ed.) (1988). *Neural Computers.* Heidelberg: Springer-Verlag.
11 Grillner, S. and Wallen, P. (1985). *Annu. Rev. Neurosci.* **8**, 233-261.
12 Haken, H., Kelso, J.A.S., and Bunz, H. (1985). *Biol. Cybern.* **51**, 347-356.
13 Hogan, N. (1984). *J. Neurosci.* **4**, 2745-2754.
14 Kawato, M., Furukawa, K., and Suzuki, R. (1987). *Biol. Cybern.* **56**, 1-17.
15 Lamb, G.L. Jr. (1980). *Elements of Soliton Theory.* New York: John Wiley & Sons.
16 Lashley, K.S. (1950). *Symp. Soc. Exp. Biol.* **4**, 454-482.
17 Morasso, P. and Mussa Ivaldi, F.A. (1982). *Biol. Cybern.* **45**, 131-142.
18 Rall, W. (1977). In *Handbook of Physiology*, vol. 1, ed. Kandel, E., pp. 39-97. Baltimore: Williams & Wilkins.
19 Selverston, A.I. (ed.) (1985). *Model Neural Networks and Behaviour.* New York: Plenum Press.
20 Soechting, J.F., Lacquaniti, F., and Terzuolo, C.A. (1986). *Neuroscience* **17**, 295-311.

16

NEURAL NETWORK MODELS FOR FORMATION AND CONTROL OF MULTIJOINT ARM TRAJECTORY

MITSUO KAWATO

ATR Auditory and Visual Perception Research Laboratories, Seika-cho, Soraku-gun, Kyoto 619-02, Japan

A computational model for voluntary movement is proposed (Fig. 1) which accounts for Marr's (*15*) first level for understanding complex information-processing systems: *i.e.*, computational theory.

Consider a thirsty person reaching for a glass of water on a table. The goal of the movement is to move the arm toward the glass which in turn will lead to reducing the thirst. First, one desirable trajectory in the task-oriented coordinates must be selected from an infinite number of possible trajectories which lead to the glass whose spatial coordinates are provided by the visual system (trajectory determination in Fig. 1). Second, the spatial coordinates of the desired trajectory must be reinterpreted in terms of a corresponding set of body coordinates, such as joint angles or muscle lengths (coordinates transformation in Fig. 1). Finally, motor commands, that is muscle torque, must be generated to coordinate the activity of many muscles so that the desired trajectory is realized (generation of motor command in Fig. 1). Several lines of experimental evidence suggest that the three sets of information shown in Fig. 1, *i.e.*, the desired trajectory in visual coordinates, the desired trajectory in body

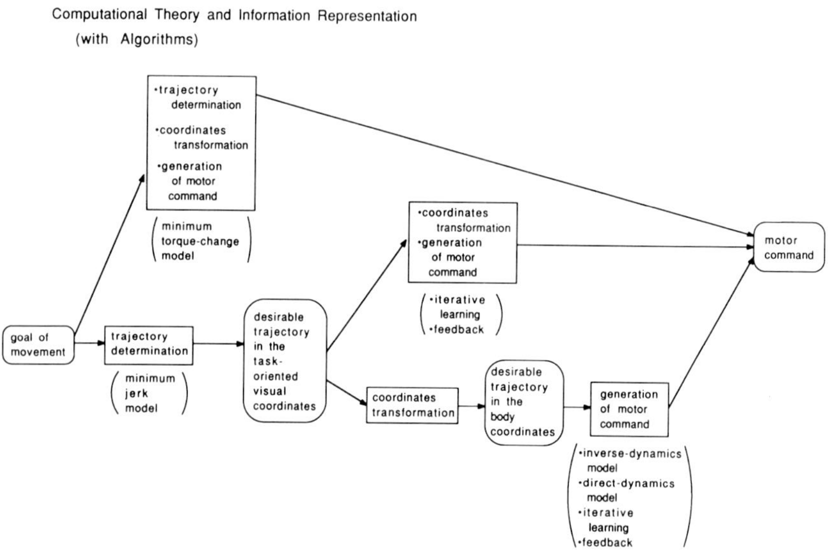

Fig. 1. Computational theories and internal information representation in the brain for sensory-motor control of voluntary movement. Computational problems are shown in rectangles. Information internally represented in the brain is shown in ovals. Possible algorithms are shown in parentheses.

coordinates and the active torque, are internally represented in the brain (*13*).

However, it must be noted that here we do not adhere to the hypothesis of the step-by-step information processing shown on the bottom line in Fig. 1. Rather, our model indicates that there are other stages of information processing which can realize the desired trajectory. In the middle line of Fig. 1, the motor command is obtained directly from the desired trajectory represented in the task-oriented coordinates, that is, the two problems (coordinates transformation and generation of motor command) are simultaneously solved. Previously, we proposed that some areas of the sensory association cortex (areas 2, 5, and 7) constitute the locus of this computation by an iterative learning algorithm (*10*). That is, the motor command is not determined immediately, but in a stepwise, trail-and-error fashion over the course of a set of repetitions.

Further, in the uppermost line of Fig. 1, the motor command is calculated directly from the goal of movement; that is, the three problems (trajectory determination, coordinates transformation, and generation of motor command) are simultaneously solved.

First, the problem of the determination of the trajectory will be investigated, and then the generation of motor command will be examined.

I. ILL-POSED MOTOR CONTROL PROBLEMS

A problem is well-posed when its solution exists, it is unique and depends continuously on the initial data. Ill-posed problems fail to satisfy one or more of these criteria. Most motor control problems are ill-posed in the sense that the solution is not unique.

We list three ill-posed control problems in Fig. 2. First, consider the trajectory determination problem for human planar, two-joint arm movement, when the starting, intermediate and end points, as well as the movement time, are specified (Fig. 2, top). There is an infinite number of possible trajectories satisfying these conditions. Thus, the solution is not unique and the problem is ill-posed.

The second ill-posed problem is the inverse kinematics problem in a redundant manipulator with excess degrees of freedom. For example, consider a three-degrees-of freedom manipulator in a plane (Fig. 2, middle). The inverse kinematics problem is to determine the three joint angles (three degrees of freedom) when the hand position in the Cartesian coordinates (two degrees of freedom) is given. Because of the redundancy, even when the time course of the hand position is strictly determined, the time course of the three joint angles cannot be determined uniquely. We note that human hands have excess degrees of freedom.

The third ill-posed motor control problem is the inverse dynamics problem in a manipulator with agonist and antagonist muscles (actuators). Consider a single joint manipulator with a pair of muscles (Fig. 2, bottom). The inverse dynamics problem is to determine time courses of tensions of agonist and antagonist muscles when the joint angle time course is determined. Even when the time course of the joint angle is specified, there is an infinite number of tension waveforms of the two muscles which realize the same joint angle time course, as indicated by solid and broken curves in Fig. 2, bottom.

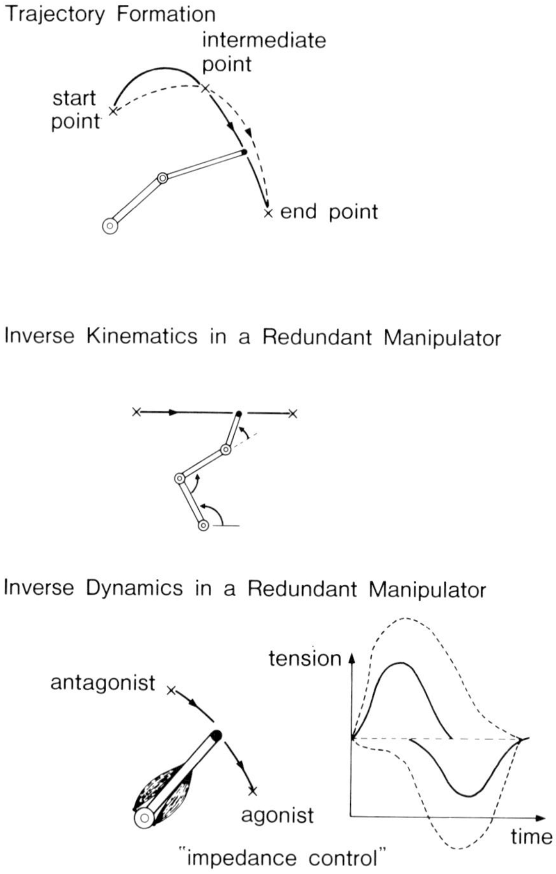

Fig. 2. Three ill-posed problems in sensory-motor control.

To resolve the ill-posedness of these problems, we need to introduce some performance index other than the above conditions which specify movement pattern. Such an objective function will be explained in the next section. This kind of objective function is still not a sufficient condition for resolving the ill-posedness. Computational schemes, algorithms and neural network models must be compatible with the objective function so that the objective function is naturally embedded into them. It is worthwhile to evaluate computational schemes and neural network models on the basis of whether they can cope with the ill-posedness inherent in a sensory-motor control.

II. FORMATION OF TRAJECTORY: MINIMUM TORQUE-CHANGE MODEL

Flash and Hogan (*3*) provided a mathematical model and experimental data which suggest that the desirable trajectory is first planned using task-oriented (visual) coordinates. They proposed that the trajectory, followed by the subject's arms, tended to minimize the following quadratic measure of performance: the integral of the square of the jerk (rate of change of acceleration) of the hand position (x, y), integrated over the entire movement.

$$C_J = \int_0^{t_f} \left\{ \left(\frac{d^3x}{dt^3} \right)^2 + \left(\frac{d^3y}{dt^3} \right)^2 \right\} dt \tag{0.1}$$

The minimum jerk model reproduces both the qualitative features and the quantitative details observed experimentally (*3*). Their analysis was based solely on the kinematics of movement, independent of the dynamics of the musculoskeletal system, and was successful only when formulated in terms of the motion of the hand in extracorporal space.

Based on the idea that the objective function must be related to the dynamics, Uno *et al.* (*18*) proposed the following alternative quadratic measure of performance:

$$C_T = \int_0^{t_f} \sum_{i=1}^{n} \left(\frac{dT_i}{dt} \right)^2 dt, \tag{0.2}$$

here, T_i is the torque fed to the i-th actuator out of n actuators. The objective function is the sum of the square of the rate of change of the torque, integrated over the entire movement. One can easily see that the two objective functions, C_J and C_T, are closely related. However, it must be emphasized that the objective function C_T critically depends on the dynamics of the musculoskeletal system. Due to this fact, it is much more difficult to determine the unique trajectory which minimizes C_T. Uno *et al.* (*18*) overcame this difficulty by developing an iterative scheme, so that the unique trajectory and the associated motor command (torque) could be determined simultaneously. That is, the three above-mentioned problems, trajectory formation, coordinate transformation, and generation of motor command, can be solved simultaneously using this algorithm. Mathematically, the iterative learning scheme can be regarded as a Newton-like method in a function space.

Trajectories derived from the minimum torque-change model are quite different from those of the minimum-jerk model under the following behavioral situations: (i) excessive horizontal free movement between two targets. (ii) Constrained and horizontal movement between two targets. (iii) Vertical arm movement between two targets (see experimental data of Atkeson and Hollerbach (*2*)). (iv) Free and horizontal movement *via* a point. Uno *et al.* (*18*) recently examined human arm trajectories under these conditions and found that the minimum torque-change model reproduced these experimental data better than the minimum-jerk model.

Since the dynamics of the human arm or the robotic manipulator is nonlinear, the task of finding a unique trajectory which minimizes C_T is a nonlinear optimization problem. The central nervous system does not seem to adopt the iterative algorithm which we proposed in (*18*). Previously, we proposed a neural-network model which automatically generates a torque to minimize C_T without explicit handling of the cost function (*11*). This network can be regarded as one example of autonomous motor pattern generators such as a neural oscillator for rhythmic movements.

We recently developed a model of a repetitive network of learning for the vector field of the ordinary differential equation which describes the forward dynamics of the controlled object (Fig. 3). The model consists of many identical three-layer network units which are connected in a cascade formation through bypath and electrical connections. The network unit consists of three layers of neurons. The first layer represents the time course of the torque and the trajectory. The third layer represents the change of the trajectory within a unit time, that is, the vector field multiplied by the unit time. The second layer is expected to acquire necessary nonlinear transformations for learning the nonlinear vector field. The output line on the right side represents the time course of the trajectory. Operations of this network are divided into the learning phase and the pattern generating phase. In the learning phase, this network acquires an internal model of the vector field of forward dynamics of the con-

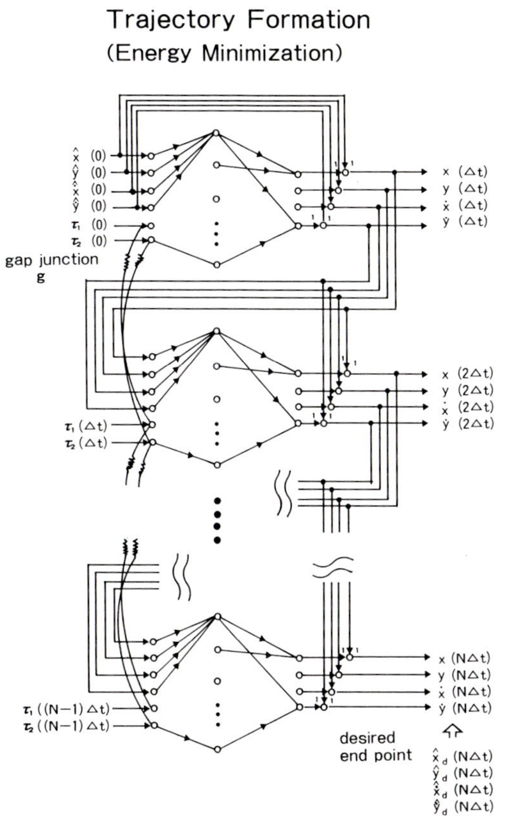

Fig. 3. A repetitive neural network model learns and minimizes energy for generation of torque waveforms which realize the minimum torque-change arm trajectory.

trolled object between the first and the third layers using synaptic plasticity, while monitoring the actual trajectory as a teaching signal. In the pattern generating phase, electrical coupling between neighboring neurons in the first layer is activated. Then the network changes its state autonomously by feedforward synaptic connections and back-propagation of errors. The stable equilibrium state of the network corresponds to the minimum energy state and, hence, the network outputs the torque which realizes the minimum torque-change trajectory. This model has several conceptual similarities with the sequential network conjoined with the forward-model network proposed by Jordan (7). We emphasize that the proposed repetitive network model cannot only resolve the trajectory determination problem but can also resolve the inverse kinematics and inverse dynamics problems for redundant manipulators (Fig. 2, middle and bottom).

III. HIERARCHICAL NEURAL NETWORK FOR CONTROL AND LEARNING

Ito (*5*) proposed that the cerebrocerebellar communication loop be used as a reference model for the open-loop control of voluntary movement. Allen and Tsukahara (*1*) proposed a comprehensive model which accounts for the functional roles of several brain regions in the control of voluntary movement. Tsukahara and Kawato (*17*) proposed a theoretical model of the cerebro-cerebello-rubral learning system based on recent experimental findings of the synaptic plasticity. Expanding these previous models and the adaptive filter model of the cerebellum (*4*), we proposed a neural network model for the control and learning of voluntary movement (*9*).

In our model, the association cortex sends the desired movement pattern expressed in the body coordinates to the motor cortex where the motor command, *i.e.*, the torque to be generated by muscles, is then somehow computed. The actual movement pattern is measured by proprioceptors and returned to the motor cortex *via* the transcortical loop. Then, feedback control can be performed utilizing error in the movement trajectory. However, both feedback delays and small gains limit the controllable speeds of motions.

The cerebrocerebellum-parvocellular part of the red nucleus system receives synaptic input from wide areas of the cerebral cortex but does not receive peripheral sensory input. That is, it monitors both the desired trajectory and the motor cammand, but it does not receive information about the actual movement. Within the cerebrocerebellum-parvocellular red nucleus system, an internal neural model of the inverse-dynamics of the musculoskeletal system is acquired. The inverse-dynamics of the musculoskeletal system is defined as the nonlinear system whose input and output are inverted (trajectory is the input and motor command is the output). Once the inverse-dynamics model is acquired by motor learning, it can compute an appropriate motor command directly from the desired trajectory.

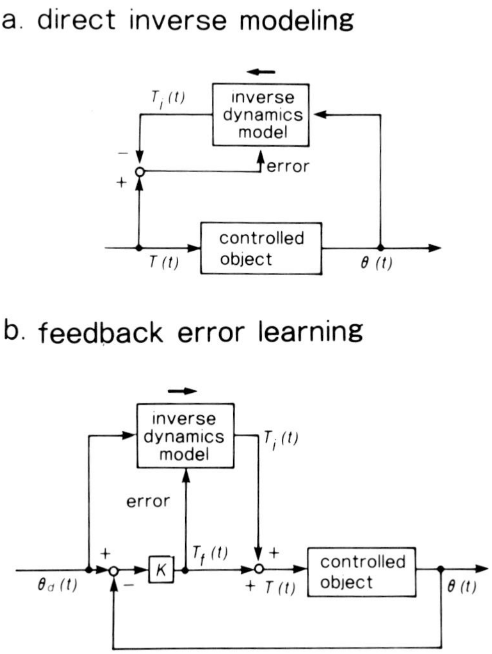

Fig. 4. Two schemes for learning inverse dynamics model of a controlled object. a: direct inverse modeling. b: feedback error learning scheme.

IV. LEARNING OF INVERSE-DYNAMICS MODEL BY FEEDBACK MOTOR COMMAND AS AN ERROR SIGNAL

The simplest learning approach for acquiring the inverse dynamics model of a controlled object is shown in Fig. 4a. In Fig. 4, the controlled object is called a manipulator. As shown in Fig. 4a, the manipulator receives the torque input $T(t)$ and outputs the resulting trajectory $\theta(t)$. The inverse dynamics model is set in the opposite input-output direction to that of the manipulator, as shown by the arrow. That is, it receives the trajectory as an input and outputs the torque $T_i(t)$. The error signal $s(t)$ is given as the difference between the real torque and the estimated torque: $s(t) = T(t) - T_i(t)$. This approach to acquire an inverse dynamics model is referred to as direct inverse modeling by Jordan and Rosenbaum (*6*).

The direct inverse modeling is not used in the central nervous system for the following reasons. First, after the inverse-dynamics model is acquired, large-scale connection changes must be carried out before it can receive input as the desired trajectory instead of the actual trajectory, while preserving the minute one-to-one correspondence, so that it can be used in feedforward control. Second, other supervising neural networks which determine when the connection change should be done are required. Third, this method which separates the learning and control modes cannot cope with the dynamics change of a controlled object. Fourth, there is not necessarily a mechanism for goal-directed learning; that is, there is no way to improve on a particular target trajectory. Finally, it cannot cope with the second and third ill-posed problems shown in Fig. 2. Jordan explained the reason for this in the many to one inverse kinematics problem associated with motor control of redundant manipulators with excess degrees of freedom (*6, 7*). For example, there are many configurations of body x_i which realize the same hand position $y : y = c(x_i)$ where c is the nonlinear function which defines the forward kinematics. "After repeated presentation of the stimulus pairs (y, x_1) and (y, x_2), the network will output a vector x which minimizes the sum of squared differences $\sum_{i=1}^{2}(x - x_i)^2$, but is not in general a solution (*i.e.*, in general, $y \neq c(x)$)." (*7*).

Figure 4b shows the alternative computational approach which we proposed and termed, *feedback error learning*. This block diagram includes the motor cortex (feedback gain K and summation of feedback and feedforward commands), the transcortical loop (negative feedback loop) and the cerebrocerebellum-parvocellular red nucleus system (inverse dynamics model).

The total torque $T(t)$ fed to an actuator of the manipulator is the sum of the feedback torque $T_f(t)$ and the feedforward torque $T_i(t)$, which is calculated by the inverse-dynamics model. The inverse-dynamics model receives the desired trajectory θ_d represented in the body coordinates, such as the joint angles or muscle lengths, and monitors the feedback torque $T_f(t)$ as the error signal.

The feedback error learning scheme has several advantages over other motor learning schemes including direct inverse modeling. First, the teaching signal or the desired output for the neural network controller is not required; instead, the feedback torque is used as the error signal. Second, the control and learning are performed simultaneously. Third, back-propagation of the error signal through the controlled object or through a forward model of the controlled object (*6*) is not necessary. Fourth, the learning is goal-directed. Finally, it can resolve the ill-posedness in the second and third problems shown in Fig. 2 because of inherence in the feedback controller.

It is expected that the feedback signal tends to zero as learning proceeds. We call this learning scheme feedback error learning to emphasize the importance of using the feedback torque (motor command) as the error signal of heterosynaptic learning.

There are two possibilities regarding how the central nervous system computes nonlinear transformations required for an inverse dynamics model of a nonlinear controlled object. One is that they are computed by nonlinear information processing within the dendrites of neurons (*8, 9, 16*). The other is that they are realized by neural circuits, and are acquired by motor learning (*12*).

Examining the first possibility, we have successfully applied the feedback error learning neural network to trajectory control of an industrial robotic manipulator (Kawasaki-Unimate PUMA 260) with prepared nonlinear transformations derived from a dynamics equation of a manipulator-idealized mechanical model (*16*). A simple training movement pattern lasting for 6 sec was elicited 300 times. Both the error of the trajectory and the feedback torque decreased dramatically during 30 min of learning. Moreover, the effect of learning faster and quite different movement patterns from the training pattern was noted; that is, the network showed the ability to perform learning generalization.

Regarding the second possibility, we (*12*) succeeded in obtaining learning control of the robotic manipulator by an inverse-dynamics model formed by a three-layer neural network (Fig. 5). In this network, nonlinear transformation was made only of a cascade of linear-weighted summation and sigmoid nonlinearity. That is, we did not use any *a priori* knowledge about the dynamical structure of the controlled object. In this study, the learning task proceeded smoothly and the network showed the capability of some degree of generalization. In this particular task, we continued to use the feedback torque command as the error signal.

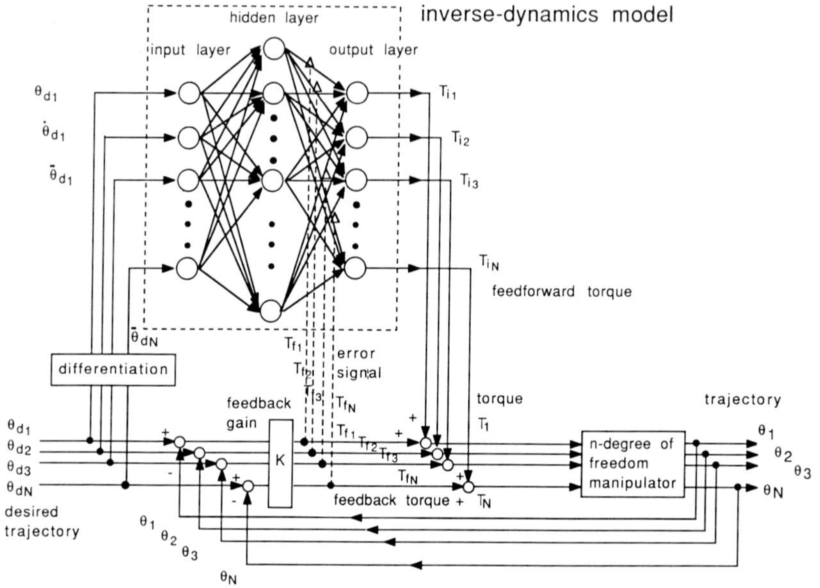

Fig. 5. A feedback error learning neural network model. The inverse-dynamics model is acquired in the three-layer neural network.

SUMMARY

In order to control voluntary movements, the central nervous system must solve the following three computational problems at different levels: (1) determination of a desired trajectory in the visual coordinates, (2) transformation of the trajectory from visual coordinates to body coordinates, and (3) generation of a motor command. Based on the physiological information and previous models, two computational theories are proposed for the first two problems, and a hierarchical neural network model is introduced to deal with the third problem. A combination of the second and the third approach was found to be very efficient for learning trajectory control of an industrial robotic manipulator.

REFERENCES

1 Allen, G.I. and Tsukahara, N. (1974). *Physiol. Rev.* **54**, 957–1006.

2 Atkeson, C.G. and Hollerbach, J.M. (1985). *J. Neurosci.* **5**, 2318–2330.
3 Flash, T. and Hogan, N. (1985). *J. Neurosci.* **5**, 1688–1703.
4 Fujita, M. (1982). *Biol. Cybern.* **45**, 195–206.
5 Ito, M. (1970). *Int. J. Neurol.* **7**, 162–176.
6 Jordan, M.I. and Rosenbaum, D.A. (1988). *COINS Technical Report 88-26*, 1–68.
7 Jordan, M.I. (1988). *COINS Technical Report 88-27*, 1–41.
8 Kawato, M., Hamaguchi, T., Murakami, F., and Tsukahara, N. (1984). *Biol. Cybern.* **50**, 447–454.
9 Kawato, M., Furukawa, K., and Suzuki, R. (1987). *Biol. Cybern.* **57**, 169–185.
10 Kawato, M., Isobe, M., Maeda, Y., and Suzuki, R. (1988). *Biol. Cybern.* **59**, 161–177.
11 Kawato, M., Uno, Y., Isobe, M., and Suzuki, R. (1988). *IEEE Control Syst. Mag.* **8**, 8–16.
12 Kawato, M., Setoyama, T., and Suzuki, R. (1988). *Proceedings of the International Neural Networks Society, First Annual Meeting*, p. 342.
13 Kawato, M. (1989). *Adv. Robotics* **3**, No. 3.
14 Kawato, M., Isobe, M., and Suzuki, R. (1988). In *Dynamic Interaction in Neural Networks: Models and Data*, ed. Arbib, M.A. and Amari, S., pp. 195–214. Berlin, Heidelberg, New York: Springer-Verlag.
15 Marr, D. (1982). *Vision.* New York: Freeman.
16 Miyamoto, H., Kawato, M., Setoyama, T., and Suzuki, R. (1988). *Neural Networks* **1**, 251–265.
17 Tsukahara, N. and Kawato, M. (1982). In *Lecture Notes in Biomathematics*, vol. 45, ed. Amari, S. and Arbib, M.A., pp. 430–441. Berlin, Heidelberg, New York: Springer-Verlag.
18 Uno, Y., Kawato, M., and Suzuki, R. (1989). *Biol. Cybern.*, in press.

17

USING ASSOCIATIVE CONTENT-ADDRESSABLE MEMORIES TO CONTROL MOVEMENT

CHRISTOPHER G. ATKESON AND
DAVID J. REINKENSMEYER

Brain and Cognitive Sciences Department and the Artificial Intelligence Laboratory, Massachusetts Institute of Technology, NE43-759, 545 Technology Square, Cambridge, Massachusetts 02139, U.S.A.

Internal models of the motor apparatus and motor tasks are useful for planning, control, and learning. This research explores a memory-based approach to modeling. In this approach models are learned by storing experiences in a memory. To make predictions the memory is searched for relevant experience. The memory used is an associative content-addressable memory (ACAM) (*11*). We have implemented an ACAM on a parallel computer, the Connection Machine (*6*). In order to explore the feasibility of the approach and identify research issues and problems, we used the ACAM to model and control a simulated planar two-joint arm and a simulated running machine.

An ACAM can be implemented in many ways. There are implementations appropriate for serial computers, parallel computers, dedicated electronic hardware, and model neural networks. We have implemented an ACAM on a parallel computer, but the issues raised and experience gained are useful in assessing many proposed memory-based motor control schemes.

I. MEMORY-BASED MODELING

This section describes how a memory can be used to represent a model. As an example, the dynamics of a one-joint arm are modeled. The model is used to compute feedforward commands for a controller. The controller combines these feedforward commands with feedback control to drive the arm along a desired trajectory. The arm dynamics are affected by gravitational, viscous, frictional, and inertial forces. The state of the arm is given by its current joint position and velocity, θ and $\dot{\theta}$. Applying a joint torque, τ, causes a particular joint acceleration, $\ddot{\theta}$. These values can be stored together as a single experience:

$$(\theta_i, \dot{\theta}_i, \ddot{\theta}_i, \tau_i),$$

where i designates the ith experience. In this study experiences are generated by a feedback controller, which commands torques according to position and velocity errors.

In order to predict the torques necessary to achieve a desired trajectory, it is useful to have a model of the arm's inverse dynamics, $\hat{R}^{-1}$, which performs the transformation:

$$\tau = \hat{R}^{-1}(\theta, \dot{\theta}, \ddot{\theta}).$$

$\hat{R}^{-1}$can be represented by a memory that contains experiences of particular positions, velocities, torques, and the resulting accelerations. Command torques can be predicted by addressing the memory with the desired performance $(\theta_d, \dot{\theta}_d, \ddot{\theta}_d)$, and finding the stored experience most similar to the desired performance. The appropriate variables of each stored experience are compared with the desired positions, velocities, and accelerations using a distance metric. A simple distance metric is the Euclidean distance between the corresponding values:

$$d_i = ((\theta_i - \theta_d)^2 + (\dot{\theta}_i - \dot{\theta}_d)^2 + (\ddot{\theta}_i - \ddot{\theta}_d)^2)^{1/2}.$$

The torque from the experience with the smallest distance, d_i, is used at each point along the desired trajectory.

This process can be implemented on a standard serial computer.

Every time a particular set of positions, velocities, and accelerations is requested, the entire memory can be searched for the closest experience. Viewed as a black box, this process implements an ACAM. The memory is content-addressable in that part of the contents of the memory, $(\theta_i, \dot{\theta}_i, \ddot{\theta}_i)$, are used to select the rest of the memory, (τ_i). In our example a position, velocity, and acceleration were used to choose an experience, and the torque from that experience was used. In the case where an exacts match is not available this process finds a reasonable answer by finding the most similar experience in the memory. In this way the process acts as an associative memory.

We have used a parallel computer to implement an ACAM. In our ACAM implementation each experience is stored in a processor of the Connection Machine, a massively-parallel computer (*6*). The Connection Machine can have up to 2^{16} processors, and can simulate a parallel computer with many more processors. Each experience can be compared to the desired experience simultaneously in each processor, and then a hardwired global-OR bus can be used to find the closest match in constant time independent of the number of stored experiences. This approach is similar to many Connection Machine algorithms that find a best match (*20*).

II. TRAJECTORY FOLLOWING

The feasibility of the ACAM was tested on two simulations, the first of which involved a simulated arm following a trajectory. The ACAM was used to learn a model of the inverse dynamics and helped improve performance of a single trajectory and a similar trajectory by predicting appropriate feedforward commands.

The arm used in the simulation was a two-joint arm (Fig. 1) with dynamics given by:

$$\ddot{\theta} = R(\theta, \dot{\theta}, \tau),$$

where $\ddot{\theta}$ is the joint acceleration vector produced by application of the torque vector τ to the current state of the arm as given by the joint angle and joint velocity vectors θ and $\dot{\theta}$. As the arm is servoed

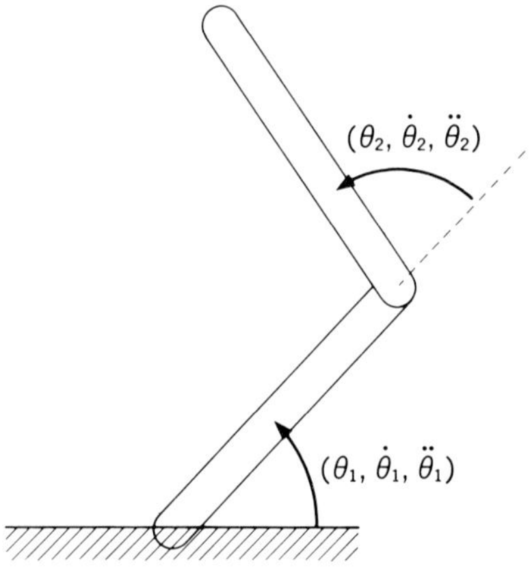

Fig. 1. Simulated planar two-joint arm.

along a trajectory, a model of the inverse dynamics is built by storing values of $\theta, \dot{\theta}, \ddot{\theta}$, and τ.

In order to use the model to calculate feedforward torques, the memory is searched using θ_d, $\dot{\theta}_d$, and $\ddot{\theta}_d$ as indices, where the subscript d denotes desired values as supplied by a trajectory planner. This search is applied before each attempt at the trajectory, and an array is filled with the feedforward torques (τ_{ff}) which are to be added to the output of a feedback controller:

$$\tau = -K(\theta - \theta_d) - B(\dot{\theta} - \dot{\theta}_d) + \tau_{ff}\,.$$

The combination of feedback terms and feedforward terms drives the arm. If τ_{ff} is poorly modeled, the feedback terms are responsible for moving the arm in a reasonable way. This is the situation when the memory has not stored many experiences: the feedback terms act as a teacher in generating the initial commands that enable the ACAM to store appropriate experiences. As the model becomes more accurate, the contribution of the feedback terms to the controller becomes smaller.

The two test trajectories shown in Fig. 2 were planned using a straight line path and a fifth-order polynomial position function which started and ended at rest and had a duration of one sec. The movements were in a vertical plane so gravity points downward in

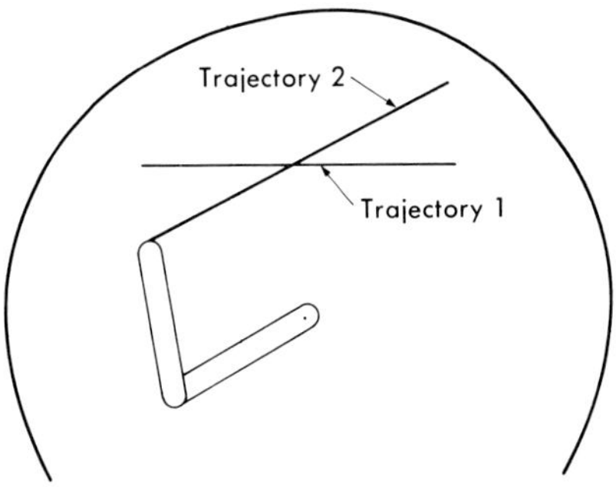

Fig. 2. Test trajectories.

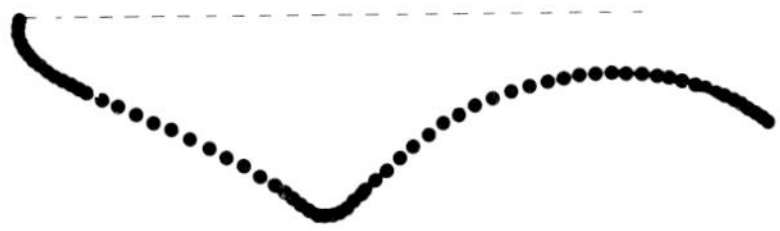

Fig. 3. Trajectory 1—feedback only.

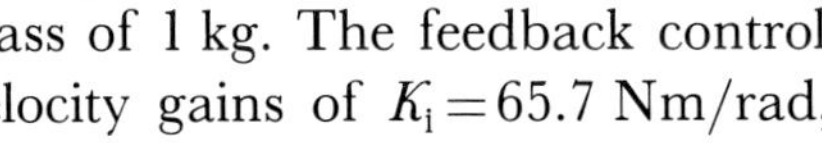

Fig. 4. Trajectory 1—first attempt.

this figure. The links were modeled as thin uniform rods each with a mass of 1 kg. The feedback controller used decoupled position and velocity gains of $K_1 = 65.7$ Nm/rad, $K_2 = 13$ Nm/rad, $B_1 = 42$ Nms/rad, and $B_2 = 8$ Nms/rad, and applied torques at a rate of 100 Hz. The equations describing the arm dynamics were integrated using Euler's method with a time step of 0.001 sec.

1. Results

The ACAM improved trajectory following for a single trajectory. Figure 3 shows the performance of trajectory 1 with the feedback controller alone. After storing these experiences in the ACAM, feedforward torques were computed using the memory. Figure 4 shows that on the first attempt using the ACAM there was a performance improvement. Figure 5 shows how closely the feedfor-

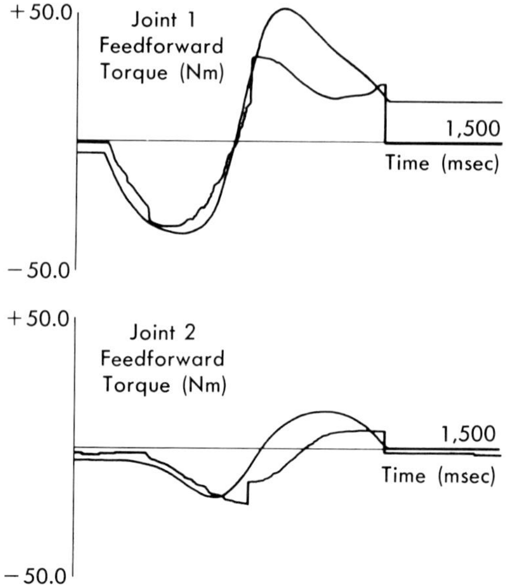

Fig. 5. Trajectory 1—feedforward torques for first attempt.

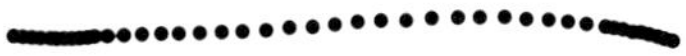

Fig. 6. Trajectory 1—third attempt.

ward torques on the first attempt corresponded to the ideal feedforward torques for the desired movement.

After three cycles of storing the previous movement's data in the ACAM and computing a new feedforward command, the performance improved further. Figure 6 shows this tracking performance, which was better than the performance on the first attempt. Figure 7 shows that the feedforward torques corresponded even more closely to the ideal feedforward torques. The ACAM built a better model of the arm dynamics.

The accuracy of trajectory following for trajectory 1 stopped improving after about six attempts. The feedforward torques for attempt ten are shown in Fig. 8, and show the best performance the

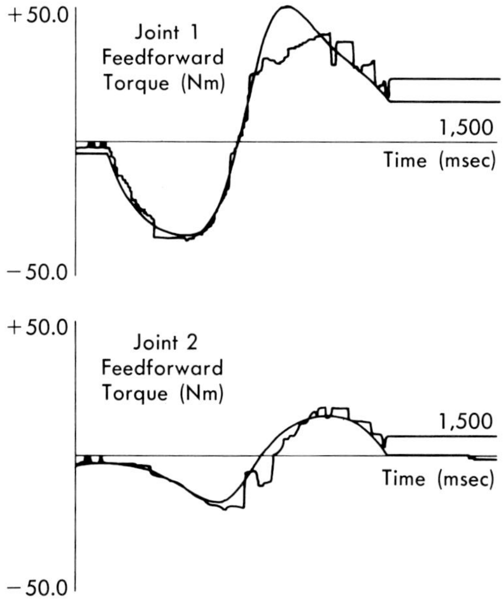

Fig. 7. Trajectory 1—feedforward torques for third attempt.

memory was able to achieve. We call this phenomena a "stuck state." The problem of stuck states is an area for further research.

The model stored in the ACAM after eight attempts at trajectory 1 generalized to a similar trajectory, trajectory 2 (see Fig. 2). The ACAM used only the experiences stored during the attempts at trajectory 1 to calculate the feedforward torques for trajectory 2. Figure 9 shows the trajectory following performance with the feedback controller alone. Figure 10 shows the improved performance using the model learned during performance of trajectory 1. Figure 11 shows how well the feedforward torques generalized from the experiences of trajectory 1. The similarity of these feedforward torques with the ideal feedforward torques suggests that the ACAM can act as a local model by generalizing from limited experience, but it should be noted that the modeling error is large for some parts of the trajectory.

The improved single-trajectory following and the generalization to a similar trajectory seen in these and other experiments demon-

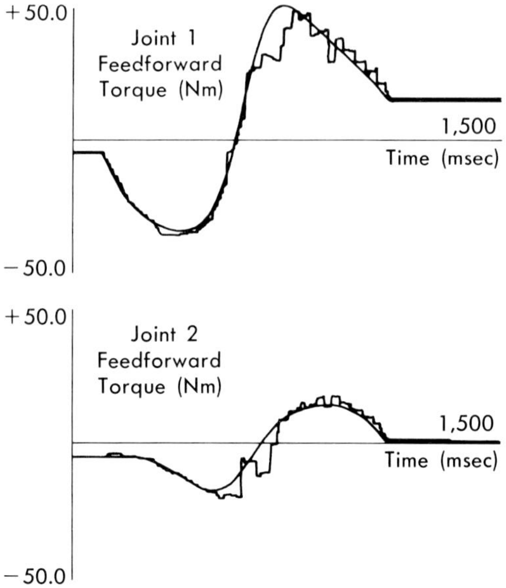

Fig. 8. Trajectory 1—feedforward torques for tenth attempt.

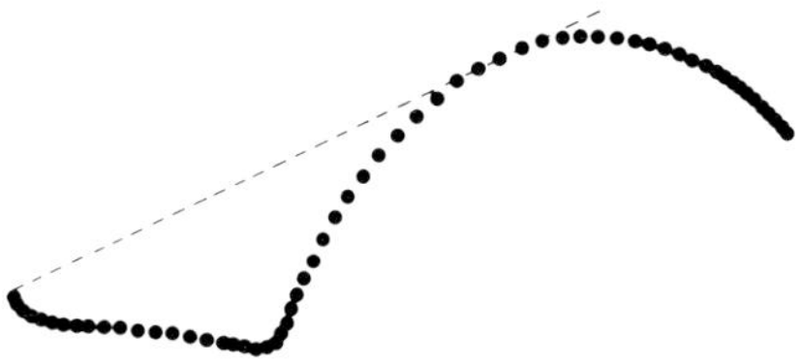

Fig. 9. Trajectory 2—feedback only.

strate that an ACAM can build a useful model of the arm dynamics. The simple distance metric was effective in retrieving stored experiences, and reasonable generalization was obtained by using the closest experience. Stuck states present a problem deserving future attention.

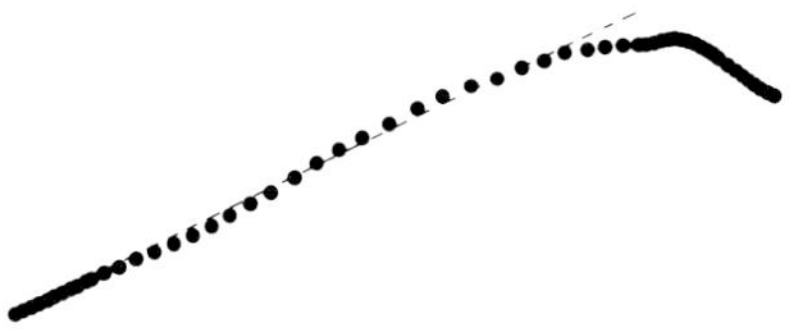

Fig. 10. Trajectory 2—using trajectory 1 experiences.

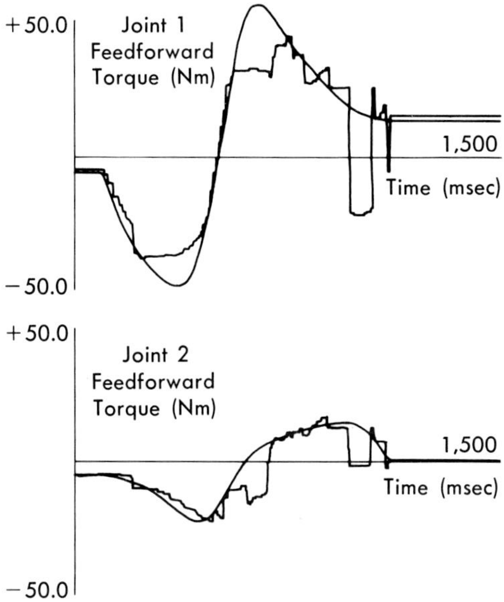

Fig. 11. Trajectory 2—feedforward torques using trajectory 1 experiences.

III. CONTROL OF RUNNING

The second simulation involved control of running. Memory-based techniques are well-suited for control of a dynamically-stable, legged system (*18*). Such a legged system is difficult to model, contains a large number of variables, and encounters only a small number of experiences (hops). In this simulation an ACAM was used to build a *correction* to a model of legged running. This learning proved useful

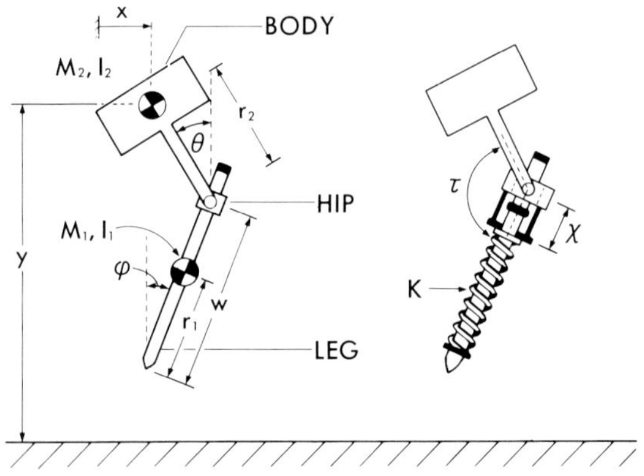

Fig. 12. Simulated planar one-legged hopper (from ref. *18*).

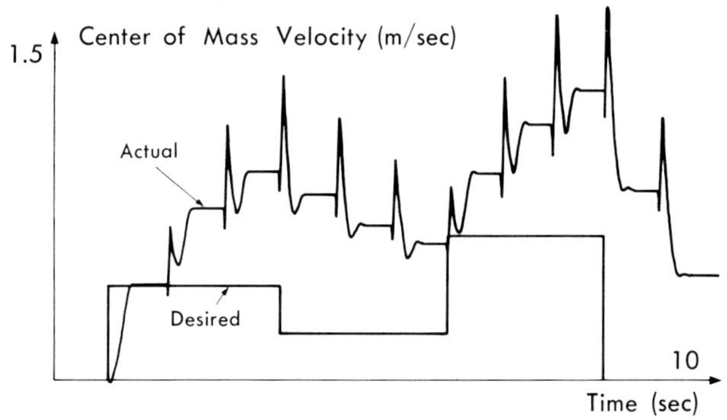

Fig. 13. Controlling hopping flight velocity—without ACAM.

in improving control of the simulation beyond the performance with the original model alone.

Figure 12 shows a simulated legged hopping machine originally developed by M. Raibert. It has a body, a springy leg, a leg actuator, and a hip actuator. Control of the hopper is partitioned into three algorithms (*17*). In order to control hopping height, the amount of energy contained in the system is adjusted by changing the length of the leg spring during stance. In order to control body angle, the hip actuator servos the body to the appropriate position during the stance portion of a hop. The hip actuator also controls balance and

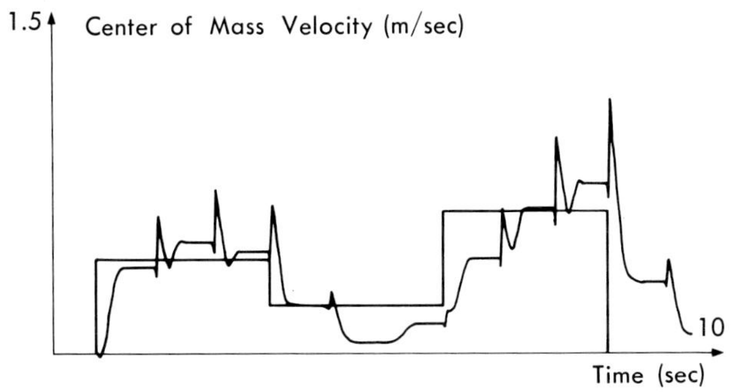

Fig. 14. Controlling hopping flight velocity—first attempt with ACAM (100 hops previously stored).

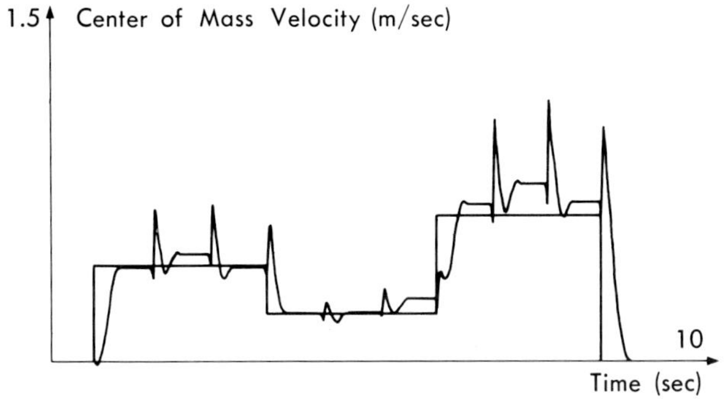

Fig. 15. Controlling hopping flight velocity—second attempt with ACAM.

running speed by servoing the foot during flight to an appropriate placement. If the foot is placed at a point called the neutral point, the machine runs with constant velocity. If the foot is placed behind the neutral point, the machine accelerates. If the foot is placed ahead of the neutral point, the machine decelerates.

The ACAM was used to improve the algorithm controlling balance and running speed. The memory acted as a correction to an analytical model of foot placement which is made by predicting the projection that the center of gravity will sweep out during stance. The projection is called a CG-print (*17*), and is approximated by $T_s\dot{x}$ where T_s is a stance duration predicted from the characteristics of the springy leg, and $\dot{x}$ is the average velocity of the machine during stance, and is approximated by the velocity at takeoff. If on landing the foot has been servoed to the center of a perfect model of the CG-print, the machine experiences no net acceleration. Thus the center of a perfect model of the CG-print is the neutral point. In order to accelerate the machine, the foot can be displaced from the center of the CG-print. The amount of displacement is dictated by a servo which uses the current and desired velocity of the machine:

$$fp_{cg}(\dot{x}_d,\ state) = \frac{1}{2} T_s \dot{x} + K(\dot{x} - \dot{x}_d),$$

where fp is the foot placement, and K is a gain.

In order to improve the CG-print model, the ACAM builds a corrective model. Corrections to the modeled foot placement are calculated in the following way. Each time the hopper leaves the ground, an appropriate foot placement for the next landing is calculated using the CG-print model and a correction from the ACAM:

$$fp\dot{x}_d,\ state) = fp_{cg}(\dot{x}_d,\ state) - A(\dot{x}_d,\ state),$$

where fp_{cg} represents a call to the CG-print model, A represents an ACAM lookup, and *state* is the state of the machine as defined by the variables $\dot{x}$, y, $\dot{y}$, θ, $\dot{\theta}$, φ, $\dot{\varphi}$, w, and $\dot{w}$ (see Fig. 12). The leg is servoed to this foot placement during flight, and the machine accelerates when it lands, resulting in a new takeoff velocity $\dot{x}_{new}$. The resulting knowledge of the actual physical transformation for this particular foot placement is used to store a correction of the CG-print model. First, a foot placement is calculated using the CG-print model, given the output of the actual transformation, $\dot{x}_{new}$:

$$\widehat{fp} = fp_{cg}(\dot{x}_{new},\ state).$$

The difference between what actually happened and what the model predicted, $\widehat{fp} - fp$, is then stored in the ACAM so that it can be accessed by $A(\dot{x}_{new},\ state)$.

Results

The ACAM learned how to correct the CG-print model and improved running performance. Figure 13 shows an attempt at a series of desired flight velocities using the CG-print model with the parameters and controller gains described in (*17*). The flat parts of the plot of the actual center-of-mass velocities are the flight velocities. Figure 14 shows the first attempt at the series of running velocities using the ACAM for corrections after having stored 100 hops whose desired velocities changed every three hops and varied randomly from −1.0 m/sec to 1.0 m/sec. Figure 15 shows the second attempt at the same series after having stored the results of the first series. Steady state errors and response time were reduced. The model that the ACAM learned enhanced the legged machine's performance. Stuck states were encountered in this simulation also, and limited the performance to a level only slightly better than that shown in Fig. 15.

IV. DISCUSSION

These feasibility studies demonstrate that useful models of motor systems can be learned by storing experiences in a memory. There are several issues that needed to be addressed in this exploration of memory-based modeling, such as the source of the experiences, how to measure similarity, and how to generalize.

The source of the experiences is usually referred to as the "teacher." The experiences can be generated in a variety of ways. For example, random torques can be applied, or a feedback controller can be relied on as a source of torques. In this work the feedback controller served as the teacher.

A simple distance metric is used to measure the similarity between experiences: the Euclidean distance between the experiences represented as points in a vector space. Even with this distance metric it was not clear how to weight or scale the different dimensions, which often had different units of measurement. How should a position be compared to an acceleration, for example? In this study the dimensions were not scaled. Other alternatives would be to scale the dimensions so that the range of values in each dimension are the same, or so that a given change in each dimension had the same effect on the outputs. Designing a perfect distance metric is difficult, but the examples in this paper show that a simple distance metric can be effective in retrieving stored experiences.

In the version of ACAM presented in this paper, only the closest experience is used, although a weighted sum of the closest experiences, or an approximation based on a curve which is fit to the closest experiences could be computed. More complex generalization schemes willl allow interpolation and extrapolation from the stored data, and may also help in dealing with noisy data, an issue not addressed in this work.

In our version of ACAM, every experience is stored. At some point memory-size limitations will be reached. To use memory space more sparingly, only the experiences which are sufficiently different from previous experiences could be stored. Memory size could also be reduced by "forgetting" certain experiences, perhaps those that have not been referenced for a long time. We have not yet implemented any form of "forgetting" or memory consolidation process.

The performance in both feasibility studies improved, but errors were not reduced to zero. We refer to this phenomenon as a stuck state, and expect it to be a problem in all ACAM based approaches to control. The teacher, in our case a feedback controller, is no longer generating improved performance over the stored performance, and only old data is used in generating new commands. Possible solutions include changing the teacher, deliberately adding random noise or other perturbations to the commands, and improving generalization and the distance metric. Model-based approaches to learning may also prove useful (*3*).

V. RELATED WORK

Memory-based modeling is not a new idea (see ref. *13* for a description of an early table-based controller). Two forms of modeling based on associative content-addressable memories are those approaches that represent the data directly, as in this study, and those that represent the data in a distributed fashion using many parameters or weights, such as in perceptrons and multi-layer connectionist or model neural networks.

1. Direct Data Representation

As mentioned previously, a standard serial computer searching experiences sequentially can be used to simulate an ACAM. The problem with this approach is that the search time increases as more experiences are added to the memory. The search time is proportional to the number of experiences. One way to reduce the search time is to use a table. The values of the desired experience are used to compute an address in the table (*13*). The dimensions of such a table must match the dimensions of the data, and therefore the size of the table grows exponentially with the number of dimensions.

A benefit of the parallel approach we have used to implement an ACAM is that memory requirements are much less than those of tabular memories. Memory size is proportional to the number of experiences encountered. It is also proportional to the size of each experience, and therefore the number of dimensions stored. The memory required grows only linearly with the number of experiences and the number of dimensions, rather than exponentially. However, the memory used is substantially more complex than a table memory. This type of ACAM is particularly well-suited for systems with a large number of dimensions and a relatively small amount of experience.

Another approach to implementing an ACAM that represents the data directly is k-d trees (*5*). This approach uses a tree data structure to speed up search for the best match. However, the number of data points that must be examined to find the best match grows exponentially with the number of dimensions in the data. Omohundro (*15*) proposed that the first experience found in the k-d tree search should be used instead, as it is probably close enough. Using this first match greatly reduces the search time. K-d trees are especially appropriate for ACAM implementations on serial computers.

An early implementation of a direct ACAM used a local representation in a network similar to many current neural network models (*21*). A single layer of neurons, each computing an inner product with the input, is followed by a maximum detection or winner-take-all network. This type of network can find nearest neighbors or best matches using a Euclidean distance metric (*10*). Steinbuch and Widrow (*22*) provide a useful comparison between network models using a local and a distributed representation.

It is important to keep in mind that all of the forms of direct data representation will give the same outputs if the design choices for the teacher, distance metric, and generalization function are the same. The question of whether an ACAM is useful for controls is independent of the question of how best to implement an ACAM.

2. Connectionist Network Representations

An alternative way to implement an ACAM is in a network (*19*). The desired experience is presented to the network as a set of activations to the input nodes. The output is represented as a set of activations on the output nodes. There may be several intermediate layers of nodes. Each node computes a weighted sum of the activations of the nodes connected to it, and some function of that weighted sum of the inputs becomes its activation. The weights are the parameters modified to make the network represent a particular function. Single experiences are represented in a distributed fashion by the weights, and each new experience may modify all the weights. Single layer connectionist networks were used early on to solve control problems (*1, 2, 23*). Some examples of recent connectionist approaches to robot control problems are provided by (*4, 8, 9, 12, 14*).

Computing the output is straightforward for connectionist networks, as each node computes in parallel a simple function of its inputs. The appeal of these networks is that they can be implemented using simple and relatively slow computing elements. However, finding the appropriate set of weights for the network is a difficult problem and usually involves some form of iterative gradient descent search, and additional hardware to implement the weight finding algorithm. In contrast, in the direct forms of data representation representing the data is straightforward. The data is simply stored without any conversion or change in representation. Finding the appropriate output, however, usually involves a substantial amount of computation with relatively complex computing elements. Stanfill and Waltz (*20*) provide an interesting comparison of a direct data representation (MBRtalk) and a connectionist network representation (NETtalk) in solving a pronunciation task.

Representing data in terms of distributed weights has several implications. The need to find the appropriate set of weights to represent a given set of experiences adds an additional learning problem to that of generating useful experiences in the first place. If an iterative gradient descent search algorithm is used to find the appropriate set of weights, previous experiences must be presented several times to the network or new experiences collected during the iterative search. Learning new experiences may degrade the representation of older experiences, unless the older experiences are stored in another form of memory and presented again during all learning. It is not certain that the search for appropriate weights will converge to a useful set of values due to the presence of locally optimum points, and it is not certain that a useful set of weight values exists. It is difficult to detect when there are no close experiences and the best match is too dissimilar to be useful. The original distribution of experiences is not represented in the weights of the network.

Although the way connectionist networks compute an output is straightforward, it is sufficiently complex to be difficult to analyze. It is not clear how to design networks to represent a particular function: how many nodes and layers are required, for example? Although successful network learning procedures have been demonstrated, it is not yet clear how well they will scale up to realistically sized problems, how effectively they use data to learn, and how quickly they can learn (*7*). The generalization function is implicit in the network design, rather than explicitly chosen. The choice of teaching algorithm is independent of the network design, and the teaching issues are similar for ACAMs implemented using direct data representations and distributed representations.

VI. CONCLUSION

This initial feasibility study demonstrates that it is possible to learn a useful model by storing experiences in a memory. The use of parallel search in the implementation of an associative content-addressable memory allowed quick searching of stored experiences, and reasonable retrieval was obtained using a simple distance metric and a simple generalization scheme. The memory was able to generalize after storing only a small number of relevant experiences. The use of search by parallel processors also allowed us to avoid many of the problems of previous memory-based or tabular approaches to modeling such as search speed and memory requirements. Further experimentation and development is required to solve problems such as stuck states.

SUMMARY

An ACAM can be used to model the motor apparatus. The model can be learned by storing experiences in the memory. To make predictions the memory is searched for relevant experience. An ACAM can be implemented in many ways. There are implementations appropriate for serial computers, parallel computers, dedicated electronic hardware, and model neural networks. We have implemented an ACAM on a parallel computer. The implementation was used to model and control a simulated planar two-joint arm and a simulated running machine. This paper describes the issues and problems that arose in this preliminary work.

Acknowledgments

This article describes research done at the Whitaker College, Department of Brain and Cognitive Sciences, and the Artificial Intelligence Laboratory of the Massachusetts Institute of Technology. Support was provided in the Whitaker College under Office of Naval Research contract N00014-88-K-0321. Support for the A. I. Laboratory's research is provided in part by the Advanced Research Projects Agency of the Department of Defense under Office of Naval Research contract N00014-85-K-0124, and the Office of Naval Research University Research Initiative Program under Office of Naval Research contract N00014-86-K-0685. Support for CGA was provided by a National Science Foundation Engineering Initiation Award and Presidential Young Investigator Award and a Whitaker Health Sciences Fund MIT Faculty Research Grant.

REFERENCES

1 Albus, J.S. (1975a). *ASME J. Dynamic Systems, Meas., Control*, September, pp. 220–227.

2 Albus,, J.S. (1975b). *ASME J. Dynamic Systems, Meas., Control*, September, pp. 228–233.
3 Atkeson, C.G., Aboaf, E.W., McIntyre, J., and Reinkensmeyer, D.J. (1988). In *Robotics Research: The Fourth International Symposium*, ed. Bolles, R.C. and Roth, B., pp. 103–110. Cambridge, Mass: MIT Press.
4 Barto, A.G., Sutton, R.S., and Anderson, C.W. (1983). *IEEE Transactions on Systems, Man, and Cybernetics*, SMC-13 (5), September/October, pp. 834–845.
5 Friedman, J.H., Bentley, J.L., and Finkel, R.A. (1977). ACM Transactions on Mathematical Software, 3(3), Sept., pp. 209–226.
6 Hillis, D. (1985). *The Connection Machine.* Cambridge, Mass: MIT Press.
7 Hinton, G.E. (1986). *Proceedings: AAAI-86: 5th National Conference on Artificial Intelligence*, August 11-15, Philadelphia, PA, p. 1149.
8 Jordan, M.I. (1986). Rep. No. 8604, Institute for Cognitive Science, University of California, San Diego, La Jolla, CA.
9 Kawato, M., Furukawa, K., and Suzuki, R. (1987). *Biol. Cybern.* **57**, 169–185.
10 Kazmierczak, H. and Steinbuch, K. (1963). *IEEE Transactions on Electronic Computers*, EC-12, December, pp. 822–835.
11 Kohonen, T. (1980). *Content-Addressable Memories.* New York: Springer-Verlag.
12 Kuperstein, M. (1987). IEEE Conference on Robotics and Automation, March 30–April 3, pp. 1595–1602. Raleigh, NC.
13 Michie, D. and Chambers, R.A. (1968). *Machine Intelligence 2*, pp. 137–152. London: Oliver and Boyd.
14 Miller, W.T., Glanz, F.H., and Kraft, L.G. (1987). *Int. J. Robotics Res.* **6**, 84–98.
15 Omohundro, S.M. (1987). *J. Complex Systems*, 1(2), pp. 273–347.
16 Raibert, M.H. (1978). *Biol. Cybern.* **29**, 29–36.
17 Raibert, M.H. (1984). *IEEE Transactions on Systems, Man, and Cybernetics*, SMC-14(3), May/June, pp. 451–463.
18 Raibert, M.H. and Wimberly, F.C. (1984). *IEEE Transactions on Systems, Man, and Cybernetics*, SMC-14(2), March/April, pp. 334–339.
19 Rumelhart, D.E., McClelland, J.L., and the PDP Research Group (1986). *Parallel Distributed Processing: Explorations in the Microstructure of Cognition, Volume 1: Foundations.* Cambridge, MA: MIT Press.
20 Stanfill, C. and Waltz, D. (1986). *Communications of the ACM*, vol. 29, no. 12, December, pp. 1213–1228.
21 Steinbuch, K. and Piske, U.A.W. (1963). *IEEE Transactions on Electronic Computers*, EC-12, Decmber, pp. 846–852.
22 Steinbuch, K. and Widrow, B. (1976). *IEEE Transactions on Electronic Computers*, EC-14, October, pp. 737–740.
23 Widrow, B. and Smith, F.W. (1964). *Computer and Information Sciences*, ed. Tou, J.T. and Wilcox, R.H., Clever Hume Press.

18

NEURAL NETWORK MODELS OF VECTOR CODING, LEARNING, AND TRAJECTORY FORMATION DURING PLANNED AND REACTIVE ARM AND EYE MOVEMENTS

STEPHEN GROSSBERG

Center for Adaptive Systems, Boston University, Boston, Massachusetts 02215, U.S.A.

I. COMPARATIVE ANALYSIS OF MOVEMENT VECTORS IN EYE AND ARM MOVEMENTS

Contemporary neural network models provide insights into some of the organizational principles that govern biological sensory-motor systems, and offer a level of computational precision that enables sharp comparisons and contrasts to be made between different sensory-motor systems. The capacity of these models to clarify, integrate, and predict behavioral and neural data is predicated upon the coordinated use of theoretical, mathematical, computational and empirical tools in a manner that reveals many more constraints on brain design than empirical tools alone. No single experimental paradigm in the behavioral and brain sciences provides sufficiently many data to uniquely characterize a neural system. Interdisciplinary theoretical and empirical approaches that can coordinate and discover both top-down and bottom-up constraints at multiple levels of behavioral and neural organization provide a much greater level of guidance towards characterizing brain designs.

The present chapter takes as its point of departure one important design principle that has been clarified by such an interdisciplinary approach. This is the principle of vector encoding that has been described, for example, in both the control of saccadic eye movements by the superior colliculus (*40, 41, 46–49*) and the control of arm movements by the motor cortex (*11, 15–18, 20, 50*).

Although neural vectors are encoded in both of these systems, they are encoded differently in each system. Why do both systems employ a neural code which, in its broad outline, seems similar, but in its computational realization is grossly different? Models of saccadic eye movements (*28, 29*) and of arm movements (*3–5*) have been developed in which these distinct types of vector coding are utilized. The models suggest that the design constraints which force these differences concern different problems of learning and coordinate transformation that are solved by the eye and arm movement systems. These design constraints are not, however, immediately evident in the neurophysiological experiments that discovered the vector codes. This chapter reviews and compares these constraints, and suggests experiments that may be used to further test the models.

II. MAP VECTORS AND DIFFERENCE VECTORS

The experiments of Sparks and his colleagues on the deeper layers of monkey superior colliculus have revealed a type of vector coding that may conveniently be called a *vector map code* (*47*). In such a vector representation, each location in a spatially organized map encodes a different vector, hence, a different combination of movement length and direction. The most eccentric locations tend to code the longest movements. Changing the polar angle of a location tends to change movement direction. Exciting cells at a prescribed location in the map tends to cause a saccadic eye movement of corresponding length and direction. Populations of cells are activated under normal behavioral conditions. The eye movement triggered by such a population has a length and direction that corresponds to the average length and direction coded by all of the cells in the population.

The experiments of Georgopoulos and his colleagues on monkey motor cortex have revealed a type of vector encoding that may conveniently be called a *vector difference code* (*16*). In such a vector representation, each cell tends to generate a broad unimodal tuning curve of direction preference that may include 180° of movement directions. Coding of movement amplitude tends to covary with the firing rate of cells in their direction of maximal sensitivity. Moreover, changes in the initial position of the arm covary with changes in the baseline level of cell activity. Thus a vector difference code does not encode amplitude and direction *via* different locations in a spatial map.

I now summarize models of eye and arm movement control in which the computation and design significance of these map vectors and difference vectors are clarified from the viewpoint of the system's total behavioral competence.

III. VECTOR INTEGRATION TO ENDPOINT AND GO-SIGNAL MODULATION IN ARM MOVEMENT CONTROL

Difference vectors are found in a model of arm trajectory control, called the Vector Integration to Endpoint (VITE) model, that was developed by Bullock and Grossberg (3–5). This model predicts how read-out of a target position command, or TPC, that specifies a desired target position, or motor expectation, is translated into a present position command, or PPC, that causes a synergy of arm muscles to contract and relax synchronously until the PPC equals the TPC. Figure 1 depicts the main variables that are computed by the VITE circuit.

Before describing these variables, it should be emphasized that such a command circuit forms only one part of the total neural system needed to control arm movements. For example, mechanisms for interaction of commands to opponent and synergetic muscles (*3*), for planning and timing the sequential read-out of TPCs from working memory (*28*, *29*), for adaptively linearizing and compensating for the variable gain of a nonlinear muscle plant (*28*, *29*), and for adapting to the inertial properties generated by variable loads and velocities (*6*, *7*) also form essential parts of the system for arm movement control.

Figure 1 shows that a TPC is subtracted from a PPC at a

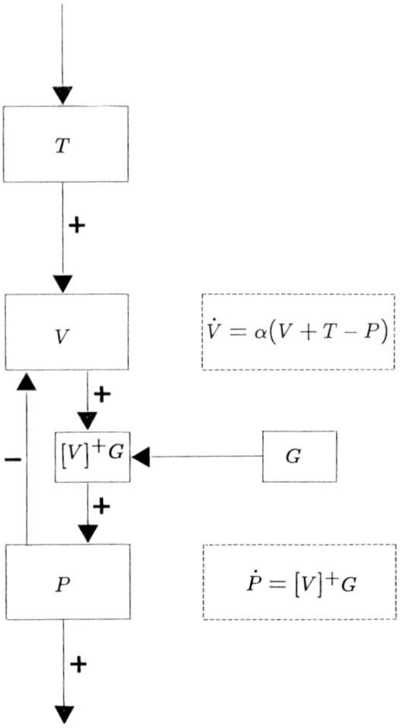

Fig. 1. Main variables of the VITE circuit: T = target position command, V = difference vector, G = GO signal, P = present position command. The circuit does not include the opponent interactions that exist between the VG and P stages of agonist and antagonist muscle commands.

network stage at which a difference vector (DV) is computed. Model DV properties are remarkably similar to data properties reported by Georgopoulos and his colleagues (Fig. 2). In particular, a large DV may be active without causing an overt movement. Such DV activation, called *motor priming*, has been reported by Georgopoulos, Schwartz, and Kettner (*20*). The next stage of the model (Fig. 1) computes the product of a DV and a GO signal, or gain control signal, that controls read-out of the movement command. The product DV × GO is integrated through time by the subsequent PPC stage. Due to this circuit design, the PPC stage generates a continu-

→Fig. 2. Data and simulation of vector cell through time: (a) Quick buildup and gradual decline of activity in motor cortex vector cells. (Reprinted with permission from ref. *19*). (b) Computer simulation of the model variables V, G, and P in response to step increment in T. Note the similarity between the graph of V and the vector cell profile (a). (Reprinted with permission from ref. *3*.)

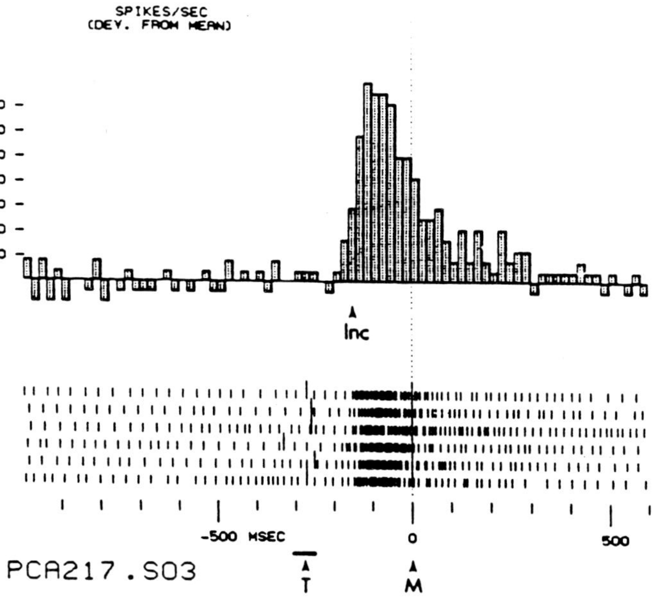
SPIKES/SEC
(DEV. FROM MEAN)
140
120
100
80
60
40
20
Inc
-500 MSEC
0
500
PCA217.S03
T
M

(a)

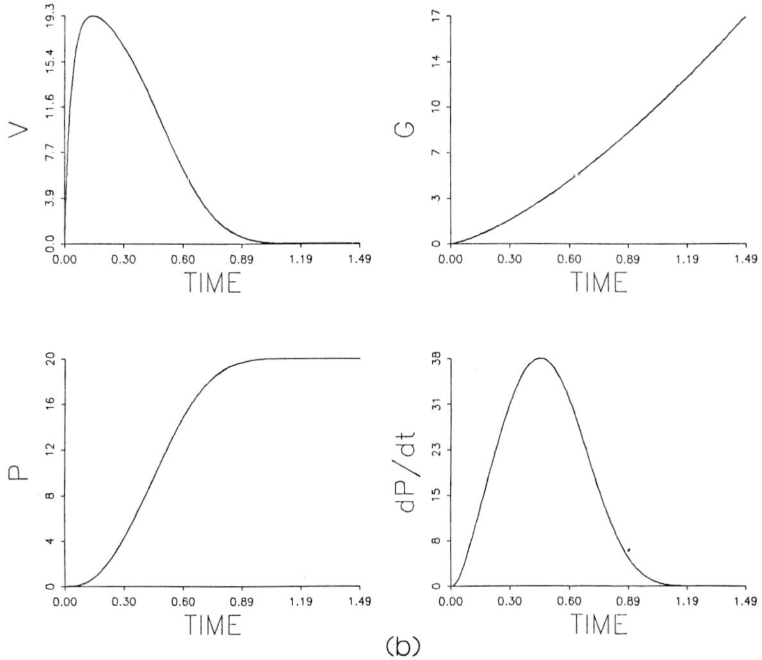
V
0.0
3.9
7.7
11.6
15.4
19.3
TIME
0.00
0.30
0.60
0.89
1.19
1.49
G
0
3
7
10
14
17
P
0
4
8
12
16
20
dP/dt
0
8
15
23
31
38

(b)

ous trajectory of synchronous outflow movement commands that gradually causes the PPC to approach the TPC at a speed that is regulated by the amplitude of the GO signal.

A large body of behavioral and neural data about arm and speech articulator movements has quantitatively been analyzed by comparison with emergent properties of the VITE model. Here, I summarize some neural data that support the existence of a GO signal, some predictions to further test the circuit's overall design, and a learning problem from which the circuit was derived.

IV. GO-SIGNAL GENERATOR IN GLOBUS PALLIDUS

Additional physiological support for the VITE model comes from recent experiments involving lesions and electrical stimulation of the basal ganglia. Data from a set of experiments by Horak and Anderson (*32*, *33*) are consistent with the interpretation that the internal segment of the globus pallidus is an *in vivo* analogue of the VITE model's GO-signal generator.

An *in vivo* candidate for a GO-signal generator must pass three tests. First, stimulation at some site in the proposed pathway must have an effect on the *rate* of muscle contractions. Second, it must have this effect without affecting the *amplitude* of the contractions. Thus stimulation should have no effect on movement accuracy. Third, this rate-modulating effect should be *nonspecific*: it should affect all muscles that are typically synergists for the movement in question.

The studies conducted by Horak and Anderson (*32*, *33*) addressed these issues. Horak and Anderson (*32*) showed that "when neurons in the globus pallidus were destroyed by injections of kainic acid (KA) during task execution, contralateral arm movement times (MT) were increased significantly, with little or no change in reaction times." This satisfies the rate criterion. Moreover, the rate of motor recruitment was depressed "in all the contralateral muscles studied at the wrist, elbow, shoulder, and back, but there were no changes in the sequential activation of the muscle." This satisfies the nonspecificity criterion. Finally, the authors also noted that "animals displayed no obvious difficulty in aiming accurately . . . they did not miss the 1.5 cm target more often following KA injections, and there was no noticeable dysmetria around the target." This satisfies the accuracy criterion.

Horak and Anderson (*33*) used an electrical stimulation paradigm instead of a lesion paradigm. They found that "stimulation in the ventrolateral internal segment of the globus pallidus (GP_i) or in the ansa lenticularis reduced movement time, whereas stimulation at many sites in the external pallidal segment (GP_e), dorsal (GP_i), and putamen increased movement times for the contralateral arm." Once again, these effects were non-specific: "no somatotopic effects of stimulation were evident. If stimulation at a site produced slowing, it produced a depression of activity in all the muscles studied. Even stimulus currents as low as 25 μA affected proximal as well as distal muscles, flexor as well as extensor muscles, and early- as well as late-occurring activity."

In the VITE model, activation of the GO-signal pathway produces movement only if instatement of a TPC different from the current PPC leads to the computation of a non-zero DV. In agreement with this property, Horak and Anderson (*33*) observed that "stimulation at sites that speeded movements did not induce involuntary muscle activation in resting animals nor did it change background EMG acticvity prior to self-generated activity during task performance." In Bullock and Grossberg (*3*) it was noted that "very rapid freezing can be achieved by completely inhibiting the GO signal at any point in the trajectory". This property of the model has also been shown to be a property of the GP system. In particular, Horak and Anderson reported that "stimulation with 50 or 100 μA at . . . sites ventral and medial to typical GP_i neuronal activity completely and immediately halted the monkey's performance in the task." Taken together, their experiments led Horak and Anderson (*33*) to conclude that "the basal ganglia . . . determine the speed of the movement."

V. FACTORIZATION OF POSITION AND VELOCITY CONTROL

The striking correspondence between the experimental results of Georgopoulos *et al.* and of Horak and Anderson and the theoretical predictions of the VITE model regarding separate DV and GO-signal processes is important because it supports the hypothesis that motor systems, like sensory systems, implement a factorization of pattern and energy (*24, 26, 27*). In the motor system, this factorization means that a movement's velocity ("energy") can be scaled up or down over a wide range without disrupting the movement's direction or terminal position ("pattern"). A similar hypothesis has recently been advanced by Eckmiller (*9*), who models it using a computationally different approach. Moreover, by using a GO signal that grows gradually during the movement time, as in Fig. 4, all synergists will complete their contractions at approximately the same time even if movement onset times of different synergists are staggered by a large amount (*3*). These properties of the model, together with the growing evidence for separate DV and GO-signal pathways *in vivo*, provide a basis for understanding how primates can achieve space-time equifinality—all synergists reaching their length targets at equal times—yet retain separate control of velocity and position. Note that rate-control models relying on *static* stiffness adjustments (*e.g.*, (*8*)) lack the critical temporal-equifinality property.

VI. AMPLIFICATION OF PEAK VELOCITY AND A GO SIGNAL TEST

Several other important automatic compensatory properties emerge from interactions between the DV and GO processes. Bullock and Grossberg (*3*) noted that in addition to compensating for muscles that begin to contract at staggered onset times, the VITE circuit automatically compensates for changes of target position during the movement time. In particular, it was shown that the model generates the amplification of peak velocity that occurs during target-switching experiments (*19*). Such a velocity amplification facilitates reaching the target after an incorrect initial TPC is replaced by an updated TPC. This speed-up occurs "on-the-fly." It is not preprogrammed, but is rather an automatic emergent property of VITE circuit interactions. It is caused as follows.

First, there is a rapid change in the TPC and thus in the DV. Then a more gradual change occurs in the DV and the PPC as the PPC integrates the DV through time. The velocity amplification is predicted to be caused by interaction of the new DV with the GO signal that was activated by the previous movement command. This prediction can be physiologically tested using an experiment that would also provide another opportunity to test if the Horak-Anderson cells in globus pallidus generate GO signals. Such a test would directly stimulate, at increasing levels of intensity, Horak-Anderson cells during a target switching task. Observed changes in movement velocity could then be used to calibrate the amount of change in GO signal amplitude caused by each level of stimulation.

VII. PREDICTION AND TEST OF CELLS THAT MULTIPLEX A CODE FOR LOCAL VELOCITY

The property of motor priming in motor cortex supports the VITE circuit prediction that there exists a stage subsequent to the DV stage at which an overt movement command is activated. The data of Horak and Anderson (*32, 33*) support the prediction that such activation may be partially controlled by a GO signal from the globus pallidus.

The VITE model may be further tested by recording from cells at the stage to which the motor cortex vector cells of Georgopoulos project. The cells at this subsequent stage should compute a measure of local movement velocity. This can be seen as follows.

These cells are predicted to compute (Fig. 1) the product of rectified difference vector $[V]^+ = \max(V,0)$ and GO signal G, namely

$$[V]^+G. \qquad (1)$$

The subsequent PPC stage computes a present position command P that performs a time integral of $[V]^+G$, namely

$$P(t) = \int^t [V]^+ G dt. \qquad (2)$$

Differentiating (2) shows that

$$\frac{dP}{dt} = [V]^+ G. \qquad (3)$$

If subsequent network mechanisms cause the arm to follow closely the outflow movement command $P(t)$, then $\frac{dP}{dt}$ in (3) provides a good estimate of local movement velocity.

Equation (3) is of great interest from a conceptual point of view. It shows that the quantity $[V]^+G$, which itself does not explicitly compute a velocity signal, *becomes* a velocity signal because of the manner in which it is transformed at subsequent network stages, in particular because it is integrated through time at the PPC stage.

The definition of this local velocity signal also depends upon the existence of a feedback loop between successive network stages (Fig. 1). This feedback loop is needed to generate movements that are goal-oriented. This feedback loop is defined as follows. Quantity V in (3) computes a time-average of the difference between P and T, as in

$$\frac{d}{dt}V = \alpha(-V + T - P). \tag{4}$$

For simplicity, consider the case when the averaging rate α is large. Then, by (4),

$$V \cong T - P. \tag{5}$$

Hence, by (3) and (5),

$$\frac{d}{dt}P \cong [T - P]^+G, \tag{6}$$

which summarizes the action of the feedback loop.

The approximate equation (6) shows that the local velocity signal is an emergent property of the entire network. It multiplexes quantities T, P, and G that are computed at three different network stages. It converts these quantities into a local velocity signal by using the feedback loop that exists between the DV stage and the PPC stage.

Given the motor cortical vector cells as an anatomical marker, it seems to be an experiment of great conceptual importance to test the existence of cells that code local velocity at one of their target nuclei. If the stage coding local velocity is found, then a retrograde marker applied at this stage may identify a location in, or near, the global pallidus. Then a direct neurophysiological test of the existence of a GO signal may be made to supplement the data of Horak and Anderson (*32, 33*). If globus pallidus cells are not marked, then this experiment may discover the true location of the GO-signal generator. An anterograde marker applied at the local velocity stage may be used to discover the location of the PPC stage. Then a direct neurophysiological test can determine its ability to time-integrate local velocity signals.

VIII. LEARNING AN ASSOCIATIVE MAP BETWEEN TARGET POSITION MAPS OF THE EYE-HEAD AND HAND-ARM MOVEMENT SYSTEMS

Our theory suggests that the VITE circuit plays two distinct roles. One role, reviewed above, concerns trajectory formation within a sensory-motor system. This role may be called *intramodal trajectory formation.* The second role concerns *intermodal learning of target position maps.* This latter role is schematized by Fig. 3. The remarkable fact is that the same TPC, DV, and PPC stages are predicted to accomplish both roles.

The learning process transforms stored representations of a target position coded with respect to the eye-head system into a target position command of the hand-arm system for moving the arm, *via* VITE dynamics, to that position in space.

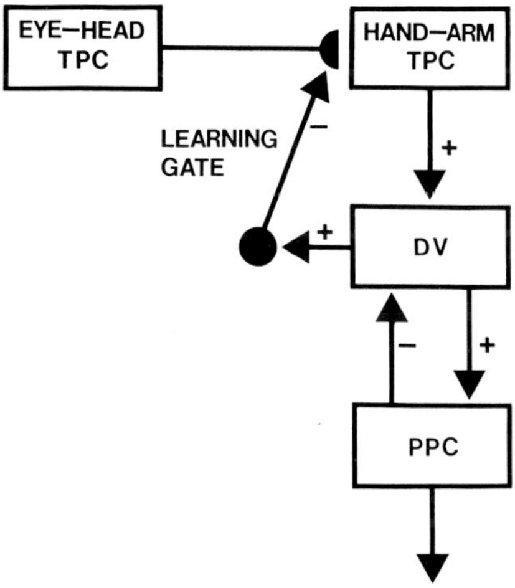

Fig. 3. Learning of intermodal transformation between target position representations is gated by the difference vector DV. This gate helps to prevent incorrect associations from being learned between eye-head TPCs and hand-arm TPCs during motor development. (Reprinted with permission from ref. *3.*)

This mapping process is of critical importance in sensory-motor control because many arm movements are activated in response to visually seen objects that the individual wishes to grasp. This transformation must be learned because, as the arm grows, the motor commands which move it to a fixed position in space with respect to the body must also change in an adaptive fashion. Our central problem is thus formulated as follows: how is a transformation learned and adaptively modified between the parameters of the eye-head system and the hand-arm system so that an observer can touch a visually fixated object?

Following Piaget's (*44*) analysis of *circular reactions*, imagine that an infant's hand makes a series of unconditional movements, which the infant's eyes unconditionally follow. As the hand occupies a variety of positions that the eye fixates, a transformation is learned from the parameters of the hand-arm system to the parameters of the eye-head system. A reverse transformation is also learned from parameters of the eye-head system to parameters of the hand-arm system. This reverse transformation enables an observer to intentionally move its hand to a visually fixated position.

Not all positions that the eye-head system or the hand-arm system assume are the correct positions to associate through learning. For example, suppose that the hand briefly remains at a given position and that the eye moves to foveate the hand. An infinite number of positions are assumed by the eye as it moves to foveate the hand. Only the final, intended, or expected position of the eye-head system is a correct position to associate with the position of the hand-arm system.

Learning of an intermodal motor map must thus be prevented except when the eye-head system and the hand-arm system are near their intended positions. Otherwise, all possible positions of the two systems could be associated with each other, which would lead to behaviorally chaotic consequences. Several important conclusions follow from this observation (*3*, *26*, *28*):

1) All such adaptive sensory-motor systems compute a representation of target position. This representation is the TPC.

2) All such adaptive sensory-motor systems also compute a representation of present position. This representation is the PPC.

3) During movement, target position is matched against present position. Intermodal map learning is prevented except when target position approximately matches present position, that is, except when the DV is small (Fig. 3). A *learning gate*, or modulator, signal is thus controlled by the DV. This gating signal enables learning to occur when a good match occurs and prevents learning from occurring when a bad match occurs.

In summary, we trace the existence of vector difference codes to two fundamental computational problems: intermodal learning of target position transformations, and intramodal performance of synchronous trajectories within dynamically determined motor synergies.

IX. VISUALLY REACTIVE MOVEMENTS AND THE VECTOR MAP CODE WITHIN SUPERIOR COLLICULUS

The type of vector map code described by Sparks and his colleagues may be analyzed as part of a circuit design that realizes a different type of learning process. This learning process enables the *visually reactive movement system* to generate accurate reactive eye movements in response to flashing or moving lights on the retina (*28*, *29*). The role of map vectors in the visually reactive movement system has been analyzed as part of a developmental sequence during which reactive eye movements to flashing or moving lights on the retina are supplemented by attentionally mediated movements towards motivationally interesting sensory cues. These movements are supplemented once again by predictive eye movements that form part of planned sequences of complex movement synergies capable of ignoring the sensory substrate on which they are built. Each of these categories of eye movement requires one or more types of learning in order to achieve high accuracy. The movement systems wherein attention and intention play an increasingly important role base their adaptive success upon the prior learning of the more primitive, visually reactive types of movement.

X. THREE INTERACTING COORDINATE SYSTEMS: RETINOTOPIC, MOTOR SECTOR, AND MAP VECTOR

The visually reactive movement system uses learning based upon visual error signals to improve the accuracy of its movements. It is assumed that a target light is chosen and stored in short term memory (STM) before a movement starts (Fig. 4). This stored representation activates a movement along an unconditioned movement pathway. The movement amplitude and direction, before learning, are controlled by a transformation of the retinal location of the stored representation into a motor representation in which the most eccen-

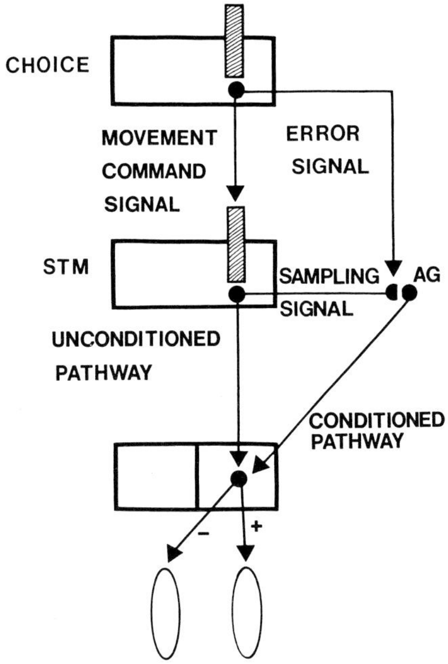

Fig. 4. A target light position is chosen for storage in STM before a movement. Its stored representation activates parallel movement command pathways. The unconditioned pathway generates a movement that may be inaccurate. The conditioned pathway reads-out an adaptive gain control signal whose size may be altered by learning. Learning occurs at an AG stage whose design is compared with cerebellar architecture. Learning is driven by a visual error signal that is activated, after the movement terminates, by the location of a newly chosen target light with respect to the fovea.

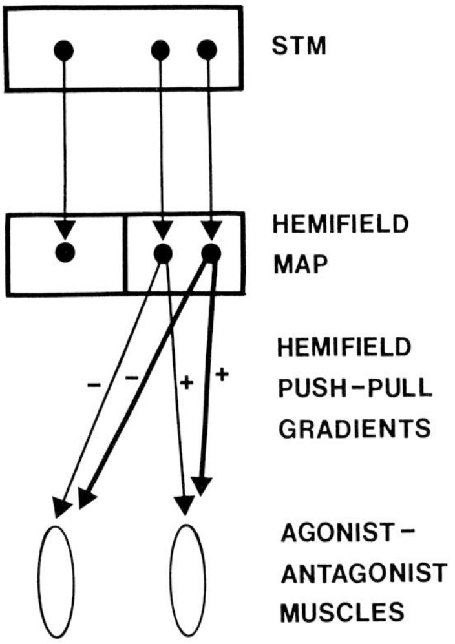

Fig. 5. The retinotopically coded location of a stored target light is recoded into a motor map that is divided into hemifields. More eccentric locations in each hemifield generate larger excitatory and inhibitory movement signals to the corresponding agonist and antagonist muscles, respectively. Opposite hemifields send opponent signals to each other's agonist muscles. When all three pairs of hemifield maps that move an eye are joined together, they give rise to a motor sector map (Fig. 6).

tric positions generate the largest movement signals. This is accomplished by decomposing the motor representation into hemifields (Fig. 5), and assuming that the gradient of connections to the corresponding pairs of agonist and antagonist muscles increases with ccccntricity (*10, 14, 21*).

The target light is stored in STM so that it can benefit from a visual error signal after the movement terminates. The stored representation samples this visual error signal along a conditioned movement pathway (Fig. 4) whose output summates with that of the unconditioned pathway to generate the total movement signal. Thus learning within this sytem controls a feedforward adaptive gain that is changed by visual error signals.

How these visual error signals are coded clarifies one aspect of why a vector map exists in the deeper layers of superior colliculus. As illustrated by Fig. 4, each light plays two roles: it acts as a movement signal for the next movement, and an error signal for the last movement. Thus the retinal location of each light must be remapped into a type of motor coordinates that can correct the full range of typical movement errors. The theory suggests that this is accomplished as follows.

XI. AUTOMATIC GAIN CONTROL OF MOVEMENT COMMANDS BY VISUAL ERROR SIGNALS: CEREBELLAR LEARNING

The theory predicts how each movement command pathway can individully benefit from visual error signals to generate a more accurate movement in the future. Its analysis leads to a model of learning by the cerebellum which extends earlier models of cerebellar learning (*1*, *2*, *12*, *13*, *22*, *23*, *25*, *34*, *35*, *39*, *42*). I emphasize two key properties of this model herein: (i) the dual action of each light; and (ii) the learning of a motor synergy. The previous section summarized the network anatomy that subserves the dual action property.

XII. LEARNING A MOTOR SYNERGY: OPPONENT PROCESSING OF ERROR SIGNALS

The second key property of the AG stage concerns its ability to convert visual error signals, which individually activate only a *single* retinal position, into correct and synchronous movement commands to *all* muscles which move the eye. Learning of a motor synergy takes place in the Adaptive Gain stage, or AG stage (Fig. 4). The AG stage is identified with the cerebellar vermis, based upon data which show that this brain region controls modification of a saccade's *pulse gain* (*43*). The conditioned movement pathway generates sampling signals which pass through the AG stage and add or subtract a conditionable movement signal to the total movement command. An error signal acts to change the size, or gain, of the conditionable movement signal. Thus, the AG stage is a region where automatic gain control of the total movement command takes place.

In order to learn a motor synergy, the system preprocesses the error signals before they can be sampled by the conditioned movement pathway. Two processing constraints conceptualize these preprocessing stages: (a) the Opponent Processing constraint, and (b) the Equal Access constraint. The need for Opponent Processing

—which is a new feature of our model—can be seen as follows.

Each eye is moved by three pairs of agonist and antagonist muscles. One pair moves the eye horizontally. The other two pairs move the eye obliquely, and together can generate vertical movements. I now indicate why an *increase* in the gain of an agonist muscle command must generate a *decrease* in the gain of the corresponding antagonist muscle command, and conversely. In other words, each visual error signal has antagonistic, or opponent, effects on the conditionable gains of the muscle commands which it changes.

In order to realize the Opponent Processing constraint, suppose that the retina is topographically transformed from retinotopic coordinates into a motor map containing six sectors (Fig. 6a). This motor sector map is an idealization that may be compared to the data of Sparks and his colleagues. Each pair of agonist-antagonist muscles —(α^+,α^-), (β^+,β^-), (γ^+,γ^-)—is represented by opposite sectors in the sector map. A visual error signal which falls within a prescribed sector increases the conditioned gain of the corresponding muscle and decreases the conditioned gain of the antagonistic muscle. This type of retinal-to-motor transformation can be used to correct undershoot, overshoot, and skewed movement errors as follows.

Suppose that a light activates the retinal position labelled 1 in Fig. 6b and thereby causes a saccade. Suppose that, after movement, the light activates position 2. Such a movement defines an undershoot error: the eye does not move far enough toward the right to foveate the light. If the error signal increases the gain of muscle β^+ and decreases the gain of muscle β^-, then the eye will move further toward the right the next time that position 1 is activated, thereby tending to correct the undershoot error.

The need for opponent processing can be seen by considering the case of an overshoot error in Fig. 6c. Here, a light to position 1 moves the eye in such a way that the error signal activates a position 2 on the opposite side of the fovea. In other words, the eye moves too far to the right. Due to opponent processing, the error signal increases the gain of muscle β^- and decreases the gain of muscle β^+, thereby tending to correct the overshoot error the next time position 1 is activated. A similar analysis shows how opponent processing of error signals corrects skewed errors, as in Fig. 6d.

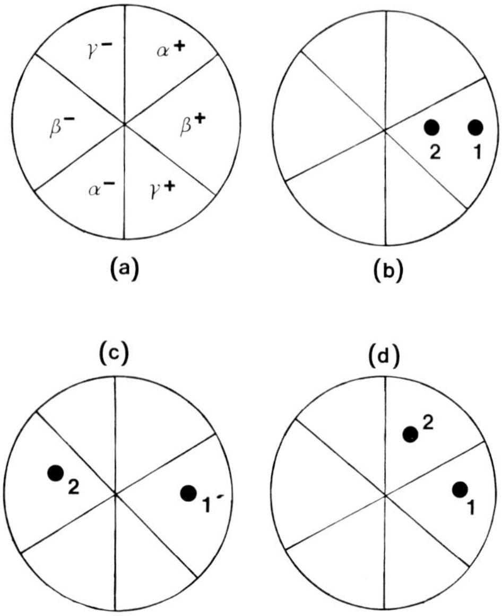

Fig. 6. Transformation of retinally registered visual movement commands into a motor sector map that can be used to correct visually reactive movement commands. (a) Retinal surface is transformed into motor sectors corresponding to agonist muscles (α^+, β^+, γ^+) and antagonist muscles (α^-, β^-, γ^-) of one eye. The text describes how the sectors convert retinotopic locations of visual movement signals and visual error signals into learned movement gain changes at the AG stage. In (b)–(d), number 1 designates the retinal position of the target light that is stored in STM and causes the movement. Number 2 designates the retinal position of the target light, after the movement terminates, that acts as an error signal. The motor sector map determines which muscle movement gains will be changed by the error signal. The sharp boundaries of the motor map are an idealization of partially overlapping motor sector regions. (b) A saccadic undershoot error. (c) Overshoot error. (d) A skewed undershoot error. (Reprinted with permission from ref. *28*.)

XIII. THE EQUAL ACCESS CONSTRAINT

Figure 6 emphasizes the fact that, before learning occurs, a light to a fixed retinal position 1 can cause undershoot, overshoot, or skewed errors. The system cannot *a priori* predict which type of error will occur as a result of its inadequately tuned parameters. In order to correct any possible error, each position must be able to activate a conditioned movement pathway that is capable of sampling error

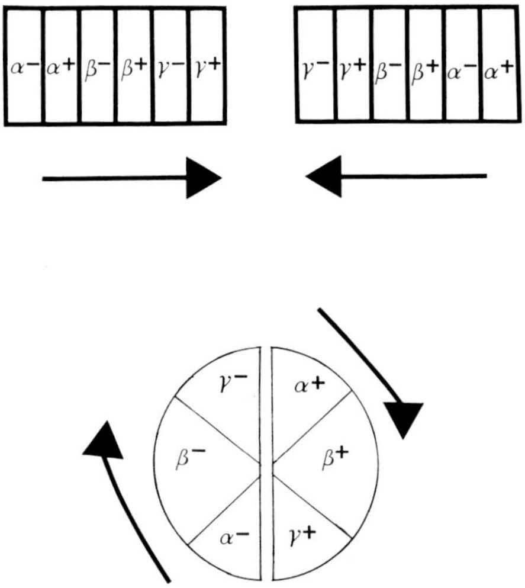

Fig. 7. Logarithmic map from sensory sectors into motor strips: each sensory hemifield (α^+, β^+, γ^+) and (α^-, β^-, γ^-) maps into a row of parallel motor strips. In this fractured somatotopy, the strips of agonist-antagonist pairs (α^+, α^-), (β^+, β^-), and (γ^+, γ^-) are juxtaposed, much as in the case of ocular dominance columns in the striate cortex. A pair of motor strip maps is depicted, one in each AG stage hemisphere. Outputs from all agonist-antagonist pairs compete before the net outputs perturb the saccade generator. This circuit works even if only agonist muscles (α^+, β^+, γ^+) receive excitatory error signals in one hemifield and antagonist muscles (α^-, β^-, γ^-) receive excitatory error signals in the other hemifield. An excitatory error signal to the α^+ strip can weaken the net α^- output of the contiguous strip *via* competition of the outputs, but cannot strengthen the α^- output signal. An excitatory error signal to the α^- strip of the other hemifield can strengthen the net α^- output. (Reprinted with permission from ref. *28*.)

signals delivered to *any* of the motor sectors. This is the Equal Access constraint, which was first articulated in a formal model of cerebellar learning by Grossberg (*22*, *23*).

In order to realize the Equal Access constraint, we have assumed (*28*, *29*) that the motor sectors are mapped, *via* a complex logarithmic map (*45*), into motor strips (Fig. 7). Then a single conditioned movement pathway can sample gain changes due to error signals which activate any motor strip. Figure 8 describes two variants of this design. Each variant realizes both the Opponent Processing constraint and the Equal Access constraint. Fujita (*14*) has also used the complex log map in his work on saccadic eye movements.

The by now classical cerebellar interpretation of this anatomy is

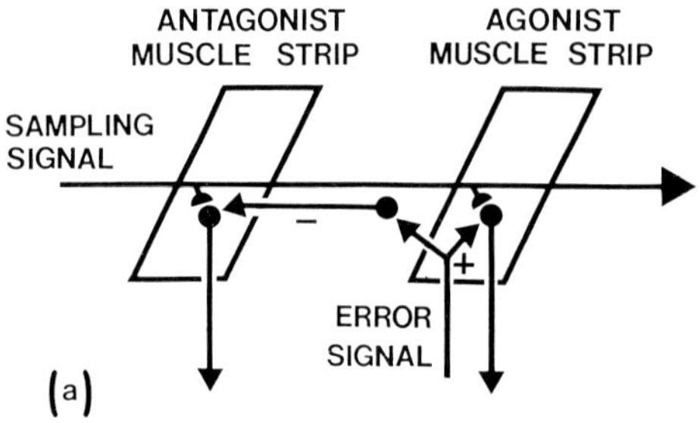

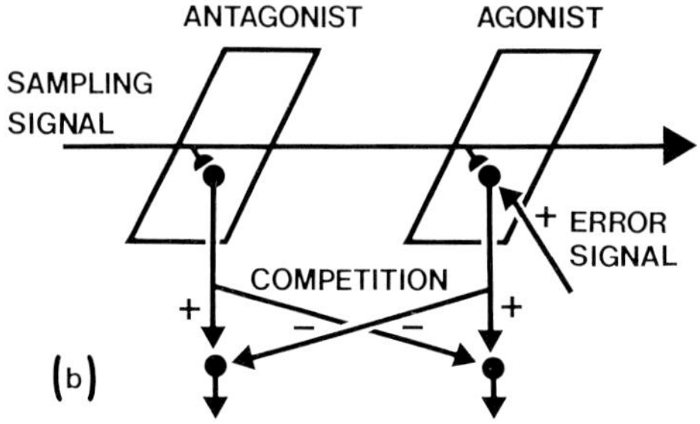

Fig. 8. Two ways to achieve opponent conditioning of agonist-antagonist muscles: (a) an error signal increases the conditioned gain at the agonist muscle strip and decreases the conditioned gain at the antagonist muscle strip; (b) an error signal increases the conditioned gain at the agonist muscle strip. Competition between agonist and antagonist muscle strip outputs causes the decrease in the net antagonist output. (Reprinted with permission from ref. *28.*)

that the sampling signals are carried by parallel fibers through the dendrites of Purkinje cells, whereas the error signals are carried by climbing fibers to the Purkinje cell dendrites (*1, 22, 23, 25, 34, 35, 39*).

In summary, visual error signals are mapped from retinotopic coordinates into motor sector coordinates and then into motor strip coordinates, so that they can all be sampled by individual movement commands within pathways capable of reading-out the conditioned gain signals to the appropriate target muscles. Such a transformation provides a simple explanation of the type of vector map described by Sparks: an increase in map eccentricity increases movement length and a change in map polar angle changes movement direction because such a representation enables visual error signals to be mapped into motor commands that are capable of correcting undershoot, overshoot, and skewed errors in visually reactive movements.

XIV. THE VECTOR-TO-SECTOR TRANSFORM: DIMENSIONAL CONSISTENCY OF PLANNED VECTORS AND REACTIVE RETINOTOPIC COMMANDS

It remains to discuss why the deeper layers of superior colliculus code movement *vectors*, rather than merely motorically transformed retinotopic commands. An analysis of this problem is spread over several chapters of Grossberg and Kuperstein (*28, 29*). Here, I outline some of the main design themes.

Perhaps the most salient issue concerns the apparent absurdity of using vector encoding when the problem is considered from a common-sense point of view. In order to compute a vector, the retinotopic location R of a light must be combined with the initial position E of the eye in the head to generate a target position T of the light in head coordinates. Let us symbolically represent this transformation by

$$T = R + E. \tag{7}$$

Then a vector V is computed by subtracting E from T.

$$V = T - E. \tag{8}$$

On the other hand, the eye moves in the head. Thus, all motor commands M must be recoded into head-coordinates again before activating the saccade generator that moves the eye:

$$M = V + E. \tag{9}$$

A comparison of equations (7)–(9) seems to suggest much ado about nothing, because (7) implies that

$$R = T - E, \tag{10}$$

so that M could have been derived directly from T without computing V at all!

The functional significance of these transformations is clarified by noting that vector coordinates V are consistent with retinotopic coordinates R, but head coordinates, T and M are not. Visual error signals within the visually reactive movement system are retinotopically coded before being remapped into a retinally consistent motor sector map. In order for head-centered, attentive, planned movement commands T to benefit from the movement accuracy that is learned using visual error signals, they must be transformed into a retinally consistent coordinate system. Comparison of (8) and (9) illustrates that movement vectors V (of the type studied by Georgopoulos!) are consistent with retinal and motor sector coordinates. Thus the head commands T are transformed into vectors V so that the vectors V can be transformed into a motor sector code. In this way, attentive, planned movements can achieve the learned accuracy of visually reactive movements. This vector-to-sector transformation converts the motor sector map into a vector map.

XV. MOVEMENT GATING, INTERMODAL MAPPING, AND COMPETITION BETWEEN PLANNED AND REACTIVE MOVEMENTS

The vector-to-sector transform is a learned transformation. Our model of how this learning process occurs (*29*) clarifies how vectors V can learn to control the movement pathways activated by a retinal position R during visually reactive movements when the vector V is derived from R, and thus $V=R$. The model also predicts how, after learning is over, a visually reactive movement to position R can be suppressed *via* a spatially organized competitive interaction (*cf. 14*) when an intended movement command V is activated such that $V \neq R$. Despite this suppression, the model explains how the movement controlled by V achieves the accuracy derived from the cerebellar gains learned by visually reactive error signals. The analysis also suggests how auditory signals (*36, 37, 47*) and planned movement sequences (*38*) can activate accurate saccadic eye movements, and how inhibitory gating of superior colliculus by substantia nigra enables planned attentive movement commands to successfully compete with more rapidly processed reactive movement commands (*30, 31*).

SUMMARY

This chapter clarifies the functional role played by two types of vector codes—vector map codes and vector difference codes—in the control of saccadic eye movements by the superior colliculus and the control of planned arm movements by the motor cortex, respectively. Vector difference codes form part of a neural network model, called the VITE model, that converts a target position command into a series of continuously integrated present position commands which are capable of generating a synchronous arm movement trajectory. The different vectors are converted into overt movement commands by a gain control signal, called the GO signal, whose generator may be in globus pallidus. Experiments concerning how to discover predicted cells coding local velocity, GO signal, and PPCs are suggested. The VITE circuit is also predicted to play a role in modulating the learning of transformations from parietal target position representations of the eye-head system to TPCs of the hand-arm system.

The vector map codes are suggested to arise due to the interaction of several subsystems of the saccadic eye movement system. A visually reactive movement system uses visual error signals to correct motor synergies that are activated by visual signals. To accomplish this visual-to-motor learning process, the visual error signals are recoded into a motor sector map. An analysis of how movement errors are corrected by this system suggest a refined model of cerebellar learning, notably learning in the cerebellar vermis.

In order for the planned and attentive saccadic eye movement subsystems to benefit from visually reactive learning, they code their movement commands into vectors which are dimensionally compatible with the motor sector code, and then transform the vectors into the motor sector code. This vector-to-sector transformation converts the motor sector code into the type of vector map found in the deeper layers of superior colliculus. The properties of this transformation clarify how auditory signals and planned, attentive movement sequences may benefit from learning within the visually reactive movement system, and how gating of superior colliculus by substantia nigra enables the competition between these several movement systems to be successfully completed.

Acknowledgments
This work was supported in part by the Air Force Office of Scientific Research (AFOSR F49620-86-C-0037 and AFOSR F49620-87-C-0018) and the National Science Foundation (NSF IRI-87-16960). The author wishes to thank Cynthia Suchta and Carol Yanakakis for their valuable assistance in the preparation of the manuscript and illustrations.

REFERENCES

1 Albus, J.S. (1971). *Math. Biosci.* **10**, 25–61.
2 Brindley, G.S. (1964). *Int. Brain Res. Org. Bull.* **3**, 80.
3 Bullock, D. and Grossberg, S. (1988a). *Psych. Rev.* **95**, 49–90.
4 Bullock, D. and Grossberg, S. (1988b). In *Dynamic Patterns in Complex Systems*, ed. Kelso, J.A.S. Hong Kong: World Scientific Publishers.
5 Bullock, D. and Grossberg, S. (1988c). In *Neural and Synergetic Computers*, ed. Haken, H., pp. 197–228. New York: Springer-Verlag.
6 Bullock, D. and Grossberg, S. (1988d). *Neural Networks* (Suppl.) **1**, 329.
7 Bullock, D. and Grossberg, S. (1989). Submitted for publication.
8 Cooke, J.D. (1980). In *Tutorials in Motor Behavior*, ed. Stelmach, G.E. and Requin, J., pp. 199–212. Amsterdam: North-Holland.
9 Eckmiller, R., this volume, pp. 173–187.
10 Edwards, S.B. (1980). In *The Reticular Formation Revisited: Specifying Functions for a Non-specific System*, ed. Hobson, J.A.. and Brazier, M.A., pp. 193–209. New York: Raven Press.
11 Evarts, E.V. and Tanji, J. (1974). *Brain Res.* **71**, 479–494.
12 Fujita, M. (1982a). *Biol. Cybern.* **45**, 195–206.
13 Fujita, M. (1982b). *Biol. Cybern.* **45**, 207–214.
14 Fujita, M., this volume, pp. 165–172.
15 Georgopoulos, A.P. (1986). *Annu. Rev. Neurosci.* **9**, 147–170.
16 Georgopoulos, A.P., this volume, pp. 3–12.
17 Georgopoulos, A.P., Kalaska, J.F., Caminiti, R., and Massey, J.T. (1982). *J. Neurosci.* **2**, 1527–1537.
18 Georgopoulos, A.P., Kalaska, J.F., Crutcher, M.D., Caminiti, R., and Massey, J.T. (1984). In *Dynamic Aspects of Neocortical Function*, ed. Edelman, G.M., Goll, W.E., and Cowan, W.M., pp. 501–524. Neurosciences Research Foundation.
19 Georgopoulos, A.P., Kalaska, J.F., and Massey, J.T. (1981). *J. Neurophysiol.* **46**, 725–743.

20 Georgopoulos, A.P., Schwartz, A.B., and Kettner, R.E. (1986). *Science* **233**, 1416-1419.
21 Gisbergen, J.A.M., van, Robinson, D.A., and Gielen, S. (1981). *J. Neurophysiol.* **45**, 417-442.
22 Grossberg, S. (1964). *The Theory of Embedding Fields with Applications to Psychology and Neurophysiology.* New York: Rockefeller Institute for Medical Research.
23 Grossberg, S. (1969). *Studies Appl. Math.* **48**, 105-132.
24 Grossberg, S. (1970). *J. Theor. Biol.* **27**, 291-337.
25 Grossberg, S. (1972). *Kybernetik* **10**, 49-57.
26 Grossberg, S. (1978). In *Progress in Theoretical Biology*, vol. 5, ed. Rosen, R. and Snell, F., pp. 233-374. New York: Academic Press.
27 Grossberg, S. (1982). *Studies of Mind and Brain: Neural Principles of Learning, Perception, Development, Cognition, and Motor Control.* Boston: Reidel Press.
28 Grossberg, S. and Kuperstein, M. (1986). *Neural Dynamics of Adaptive Sensory-motor Control: Ballistic Eye Movements.* Amsterdam: Elsevier/North-Holland.
29 Grossberg, S. and Kuperstein, M. (1989). *Neural Dynamics of Sensory-motor Control*, Expanded Edition. Elmsford, N.Y.: Pergamon Press.
30 Hikosaka, O., this volume, pp. 101-109.
31 Hikosaka, O. and Wurtz, R.E. (1983) *J. Neurophysiol.* **49**, 1268-1284.
32 Horak, F.B. and Anderson, M.E. (1984a). *J. Neurophysiol.* **52**, 290-304.
33 Horak, F.B. and Anderson, M.E. (1984b). *J. Neurophysiol.* **52**, 305-322.
34 Ito, M. (1974). In *The Neurosciences, Third Study Program*, ed. Schmidt, F.O. and Worden, F.G., Cambridge, MA: MIT Press.
35 Ito, M. (1984). *The Cerebellum and Neural Control.* New York: Raven Press.
36 Knudsen, E.I. (1984). *Trends Neurosci.*, **7**, 326-330.
37 Konishi, M. (1984). In *Comparative Physiology of Sensory Systems*, ed. Bolis, L., Keynes, R.D., and Maddrell, S.H.P. Cambridge: Cambridge University Press.
38 Kowler, E. (1982). Characteristics and visual consequences of saccades used to scan displays. Presentation at AFOSR Technical Meeting, Sarasota, Florida.
39 Marr, D. (1969). *J. Physiol. (London)* **202**, 437-470.
40 Mays, L.E. and Sparks, D.L. (1980). *Science* **208**, 1163-1165.
41 Mays, L.E. and Sparks, D.L. (1981). In *Progress in Oculomotor Research*, ed. Fuchs, A.F. and Becker, W., pp. 39-47. New York: Elsevier/North-Holland.
42 McCormick, D.A. and Thompson, R.F. (1984). *Science* **223**, 296-299.
43 Optican, L.M. and Robinson, D.A. (1980). *J. Neurophysiol.* **44**, 1058-1076.
44 Piaget, J. (1963). *The Origins of Intelligence in Children.* New York: Norton.
45 Schwartz, E.L. (1980). *Vision Res.* **20**, 645-669.
46 Sparks, D.L. (1978). *Brain Res.* **156**, 1-16.
47 Sparks, D.L., this volume, pp. 125-136.
48 Sparks, D.L. and Jay, M. (1987). In *Vision, Brain, and Cooperative Computation*, ed. Arbib, M.A. and Hanson, A.R., pp. 109-128. Cambridge, MA: MIT Press.
49 Sparks, D.L. and Mays, L.E. (1981). In *Progress in Oculomotor Research*, ed. Fuchs, A.F. and Becker, W. New York: Elsevier/North-Holland.
50 Tanji, J. and Evarts, E.V. (1976). *J. Neurophysiol.* **39**, 1062-1068.

SUBJECT INDEX

AUTHOR INDEX